ACPL ITEM
DISCARDED

MULTI-COUNTY PUBLIC LIBRARY

3 1833 01422 6353

DEC 19 '77

Dr. Kugler's Seven Keys to a Longer Life

DR. HANS J. KUGLER

STEIN AND DAY/*Publishers*/New York

First published in 1978
Copyright © 1978 by Hans Kugler
All rights reserved
Printed in the United States of America
Stein and Day/*Publishers*/Scarborough House,
Briarcliff Manor, N.Y. 10510

Library of Congress Cataloging in Publication Data

Kugler, Hans J.
    Dr. Kugler's Seven Keys to a Longer Life

    Includes bibliographical references.
    1. Aging. 2. Longevity. 3. Gerontology.
I. Title. II. Title: Seven keys to a longer life.
QP86.K83   613'.04'38   77-3014
ISBN 0-8128-2267-6

Acknowledgments

1983406

For their excellent work in editing, and for their patience in incorporating the latest research findings into this manuscript, I would like to express my thanks to Ms. Michaela Hamilton and Mr. Joshua Stein of the Stein and Day editorial staff.

As one goes through life, on rare occasions one meets great people who not only stand out as experts in their fields of professional work, but who also, due to their personalities and beliefs in what they are doing, have affected one's life in so positive a way that one is very proud and honored to have known them. Some of these people in my life were:

Carlton Fredericks
Eberhard Schmid
Georg Strocka
Fausto Ramirez
Richard Passwater
Virginia Livingston
David N. Smith
Richard O. Brennan

ACKNOWLEDGMENTS

My special thanks also go to the many researchers in gerontology who, in spite of under-financing, patiently continue their work. Without their efforts this book would not have been possible.

Contents

CONTENTS

Introduction

Two years ago, I visited some friends in the New York sub-
urbs. Everyone in the family seemed uptight, as if each wanted
to tell me something but was afraid to. The 19-year-old
daughter mentioned her grandmother, who traveled a lot
during semester breaks. Semester breaks? Well, the daughter
explained, the grandmother had some friends who went to
college. . . . But we were interrupted when her father asked
us to come into the dining room for supper.

The conversation remained friendly during the meal, but
something was in the air. After dinner, the father invited me
into his study for a cognac. There, he finally told me what was
bothering everyone. Grandmother was coming for a short
visit. She was the black sheep of the family because she had
a young boyfriend who was in college. Whenever there was
a semester break, she would pick him up and go traveling with
him. She had enough money, and he was nuts about her.

It grew later and later, but grandmother hadn't shown up,
so we all went to bed. At about 5 o'clock in the morning I
woke up to go to the bathroom. When I opened the door, I
saw a naked woman standing in front of the sink, washing
herself. Since she hadn't seen me, I quietly moved to close the

1

door. Then I realized that nobody I had met in this family was that good looking. I opened the door again, just a bit, and took a closer look at a gorgeous woman. Her graceful body could turn on any man. From her face, which appeared to be both young and old at the same time, I could tell that she must be the grandmother about whom my friends had been telling me. "Sensuous" was the best way to describe her.

I went back to bed and, later in the morning, met her formally. She was magnificent: open-minded, well educated, and adept at making a new acquaintance feel like an old friend. Earlier in her life, she had been involved in getting women into sports, and since then had kept active as a swimmer and jogger. She had the vigor of many people half her age, and seemed to get a great deal of enjoyment out of life.

Charles Degan, in his book *Age Without Fear,* mentions several better-known examples of older people who have fought the effects of aging successfully. Winston Churchill wrote a magnificent 6-volume history of World War II in his late 70s and won the Nobel Prize in literature for his accomplishment. Dr. Lillien Martin learned to roller-skate at 80 and managed a large cooperative farm for oldsters at 89. Benjamin Franklin wrote his remarkable autobiography after his eightieth year, and Grandma Moses, at 78, decided to start painting. Degan himself says:

> "At eighty-eight, this I know: it is possible to age successfully. It is possible, with knowledge, faith and courage, to build against the declining years a fine and sturdy house. Build this house, and your age will be, as Shakespeare truly said, 'as a lusty winter, frosty but kindly'."

These healthy, active oldsters are not special people. In fact, they are not much different from you and me. We all have the potential to be as vigorous as a Churchill, as prolific as

2

Grandma Moses, if we follow the right health habits and take reasonable precautions in our lifestyles. Naturally, the person who establishes healthy patterns early in life can expect better results than the person who starts later, but it's never too late. Researchers have shown that even the elderly can feel and look younger within a short time.

Aging research is a relatively new science that includes the efforts of doctors, technicians, biologists, chemists, and other specialists around the world. New discoveries are being published continuously in professional journals, and our understanding of the aging process increases every month. By applying our present knowledge in the various areas of aging research, life extensions of up to 100 percent—double the normal expectancy—have been achieved in recent studies.

In addition, a new area of aging research is being explored with a large degree of success. A few years ago, in a speech before the International Academy of Preventive Medicine, I speculated on the presence of a "center of aging" in the brain. It has now been confirmed that this center in the brain can be stimulated to send out messages—we might call them "youth signals"—to keep the various organ systems functioning at their peak efficiency levels.

It is safe to say that all of us could increase our life expectancies by heeding the lessons to be learned from current aging research. Many of us could lengthen our lifespans by as much as 35 to 40 years. Perhaps the best part of the picture is that, as we take the proper steps toward a longer life, we will be preventing diseases and keeping our bodies and minds in good shape so we can, to paraphrase Dr. Irene Gore, "add years to our lives and life to our years."

Where should you start, and how far can you go? Only you yourself will be able to answer these questions. Youthful change depends upon how much you truly want to stay physically fit, mentally alert, younger looking, and sexually active.

3

It also depends on how much you are willing to do to achieve the results you want.

As a gerontologist, I often have the feeling that people expect scientists to come up with a pill that will make them younger, more attractive, intelligent, and energetic without requiring one iota of personal effort. Remember, you are what you want to be. The more strongly you want something and are willing to work for it, the more likely you are to get it. We are all too ready to blame our genes, the environment, our jobs, our partners in love, the government, and the economic situation for keeping us from what we want to achieve. True, all these factors, and many others, affect the aging process of any individual. But what is important above all is the fact that we can delay aging and prevent diseases if we so desire.

The purpose of this book is to help you live longer and better by acquainting you with the most recent findings in the field of aging research, and by helping you to incorporate those findings into your lifestyle. A few of the treatments described here are not available in the United States because they have not yet been approved by the Food and Drug Administration (FDA). Many observers, myself included, believe that in its attempt to keep harmful substances from reaching the American public, the FDA unnecessarily withholds many valuable drugs from distribution. My intention is to inform you as to which medications have been used effectively and are available in other countries so that you can ask your doctor about them, follow their coverage in the news media, and decide for yourself whether to pursue them.

Dr. Bernard L. Strehler, of the University of Southern California, said in 1974, "With even moderate funding, the key gerontological questions should yield within the next five years or less." Many of those questions are now answered or are on the verge of being answered. There is much we can do to improve our chances of living a long and rewarding life. Hopefully this book will provide the starting point.

In case there are specific subjects you want to study further, I have included an extensive set of notes at the back of the book. The publications referred to in the notes range from books for the general reader to journal articles intended for professionals.

Part I

Understanding Aging

"In all my autopsies (and I have performed quite a few), I have never seen a man who died of old age."

Dr. Hans Selye
Stress Without Distress

Chapter 1

Beyond the Average Lifespan

The average human lifespan in the
United States is about 70 years.

The oldest man in modern times,
Shirali Mislimov, died in 1975 at 168.

According to your chronological age you may be 20 or 60,
50 or 90, but your real age is determined by the state of the
cells in your body. Both your external appearance and your
physical performance are related to the degree to which your
internal cells have aged. Research has recently demonstrated
that, to a great extent, we have it in our power to control this
aging process.

There are many factors that can affect an individual's rate
of aging, and many people tend to lump them together as
"old age." Professor Hans Selye, in his book *Stress Without
Distress,* states:

"What makes me so certain that the human life span is
far in excess of the actual one is this: among all my autopsies (and I have performed quite a few), I have never seen
a man who died of old age. In fact, I do not think anyone

9

has ever died of old age yet. We invariably die because one vital part has worn out too early in proportion to the rest of the body."

The fact is that the various parts of the body do not age at the same speed. For example, the average brain attains its maximum weight during the second decade of life, the spleen during the third, and the bone structure during the fourth. Muscles and the liver tend to be heaviest during the fifth decade, while the heart and lungs usually attain their greatest weights during the eighth decade of life. These findings represent "the norm," an average cross-section of different people. But does such a cross-section really tell us what is normal for any one individual?

The Average Lifespan

Dr. Roger Williams, a noted nutrition expert, has devoted a great deal of study to the question of what is average for a group of people as opposed to what is normal for an individual. In attempting to establish daily requirements in respect to nutrients and vitamins, Dr. Williams became convinced that "the average person" doesn't really exist. Nutritional requirements are so different that if you, the reader, were to take in the "minimum daily required" foods, you would probably be deficient or over-fed in several of the basic nutrients.

Experiments in the field of aging research have led scientists to a similar conclusion: The so-called "average" lifespan of 70 years is not necessarily the normal one for any given individual. Nor should it be considered the maximum.

A HYPOTHETICAL EXPERIMENT

Let's say it is a Friday night. We'll go to a neighborhood bar and pick out a group of middle-aged businessmen, which we'll call "Group A." Then we'll go a few blocks down the road to a health club and pick out another group of businessmen of approximately the same ages. These we'll call "Group B."

We encourage those in Group A to continue their poor health habits and those in Group B to continue their healthy routines. But we also monitor Group B's blood analysis, give them appropriate instructions, and from time to time send them abroad for some additional treatments.

For the sake of the experiment, let's assume we keep track of these people for about 40 years and that we constantly measure the effectiveness of their organs and various systems. It is highly improbable that we shall find the same changes between ages 35 and 75 in both groups.

Who is "average?"

There are several areas in this world, including the high peaks of the Andes in Peru and the Ukraine in the USSR, where people grow to be very old. The oldest man known, Shirali Mislimov, reached the age of 168. Ages between 120 and 130 are not unusual in some regions, and these long-lived people remain alert and very active. In fact, we find examples of successful aging if we just turn on the TV and watch the Senior Olympics.

It is no longer a secret why these people stay youthful as they advance in years. When we check what all these people have in common, we find they all shared some very basic rules which researchers in the health field and gerontology have been advocating for a long time. As Professor Dmitry Chebotarev, head of the Russian Department of Gerontology, says, "Brain and muscles age least if used most." So why are we sitting here doing nothing?

11

In discussing the aging process in any one individual, one thing is certain: The natural human lifespan can differ vastly from the norm. For this reason no one needs to feel trapped by the aging statistics of the population at large as presented to us by the "experts" in this field.

The Seven Essential Life Factors

When people ask me how they can live a longer and healthier life, I usually begin by warning them they may have to completely restructure their habits and lifestyles. Then, if they agree that changes are worthwhile in order to stay physically fit, mentally alert, younger looking, and sexually active, and possibly even reverse some of the effects of their aging process, I tell them about the seven essential life factors that are explained in Part II of this book.

Our total approach for a healthier and longer life will require some changes and cooperation on your part. To put it bluntly, programs that promise eternal youth through "five minutes of exercise per day" or "one injection per month" just don't work. These gimmicks on the market with their shortcuts to happiness only guarantee one thing: to drain your pocketbook.

Fortunately, the available findings in this area indicate we don't have to be perfect. We can make our changes in ways that will be fun instead of work. The rewards are tremendous: Besides improving our health in general we will also prevent major diseases like cancer, heart attack, hypoglycemia, diabetes, and emphysema.

What I will do in this book is to explain why you should do certain things and how they work. Once you have a better understanding of the functioning of your body, you can evaluate yourself in relation to the new methods and predict how well they will work for you.

First, let's take stock of your situation. What is your current state of health? Are you already following some of the routines suggested for extending your lifespan? How long can you expect to live if you continue your current habits?

The following quiz was designed to measure your expected longevity. Answer the questions honestly and carefully, then examine the number you come up with. Are you satisfied with it? Would you like to raise it? If so, this book can help you. After you've read it, you may want to return to this section and take the longevity quiz again. You may get dramatically different results the second time!

The Longevity Quiz

Numerous factors affect your life expectancy. In some cases the degree of influence is known and in others it can be estimated. Keep in mind that the outcome of the following quiz, due to its estimated variables and your biochemical individuality, does not predict your exact life expectancy. It should merely serve as an aid for your health approach.

We'll start with the number 25: Add or subtract   25
points as indicated below.

Heredity:

Women only: add 2 points   2
For each parent who lived past 75: add 1 point   1
For each parent who lived past 80: add 1 more
point   1
If *both* parents have lived past 80: add 1 point   1

13

If one or both parents are still alive:

For each grandparent who lived past 75: add 1 point   —

For each parent who is in excellent health (no heart disease, cancer, respiratory disease; normal weight; active): add 1 point   —

For each parent in bad health: subtract 1 point   —

Distress:

At work, if the stress level is low: add 1 point   —

In your personal life, if the stress level is low: add 1 point   —

If you can honestly say that you know how to handle stress and that it doesn't affect your life: add 1 point   —

Nutrition:

If you eat regular meals, don't skip breakfast: add 1 point   —

If you keep sugar and refined carbohydrates low: add 1 point   —

If you keep fats (butter, margarine, animal fats, etc.) very low: add 2 points   —

If you prefer fresh, quality foods: add 1 point   —

If you frequently eat junk foods and stop at quick food stands: subtract 2 points   —

If you buy at least some high-quality foods in your health food store: add 1 point   —

If you read the label when you go food shopping and stay away from additives as much as possible: add 1 point   —

Your weight:

If you are slim and trim, perfect weight: add 2
points ___

If you are 5—10 pounds overweight: subtract 1
point ___

If you are more than 10 pounds overweight:
subtract 1 point ___

If you are more than 20 pounds overweight:
subtract 1 point ~1

Exercise:

If you have a regular exercise program: add 1
point 1

If it includes an endurance exercise like jogging or
long-distance swimming: add 2 points ___

If you don't exercise regularly: subtract 2 points ___

If you have a regular program of physical therapy,
massages, etc.: add 1 point ___

If you make sure to warm up and cool down when
exercising: add 1 point 1

Smoking cigarettes:

If you don't smoke: add 6 points 6

For every 15 years smoked: subtract 1 point ___

If you spend appreciable time inhaling other
people's cigarette smoke (in closed rooms with
them): subtract 1 point ___

If you smoke up to one pack per day: subtract 2
points ___

If you smoke more than one pack per day: subtract
4 points ___

If you smoke, but make an attempt to smoke low tar and nicotine and filter cigarettes: add 1 point ___

Air and water:

If you work and live in clean air: add 1 point _1_
If you work in polluted air: subtract 1 point ___
If you live in polluted air: subtract 1 point ___
If air purifiers are installed where the pollution is high: add 1 point ___
If you use good well water for drinking and cooking: add 1 point ___
If you drink commercial distilled water: subtract 1 point
If you drink tap water: subtract 1 point _−1_

Financial security:

If you have a personal retirement or investment program to assure financial independence after retirement: add 2 points _2_
If, in the event of an emergency, or after retirement, you will have to rely solely on social security: subtract 3 points ___
Would a minor crisis, such as the loss of a job, illness, etc. put you under serious financial stress? If yes: subtract 1 point ___

Vitamin and mineral intake:
If you take a multivitamin and mineral formulation: add 2 points _2_
If you take some extra vitamin C: add 1 point _1_
If you take some extra vitamin E: add 1 point _1_
If you are a woman using birth control pills, do you take extra B-vitamins? If yes: add 1 point ___

16

Do you know what your calcium, phosphorus, and magnesium intake from foods alone is? If yes: add 1 point _/_

Do you take additional larger amounts of minerals without having established the need for them through a nutrition evaluation? If yes: subtract 1 point ___

Do you use other healthy foods like brewer's yeast, liver tablets, wheat germ, sprouts, etc.? If yes: add 1 point _/_

Lifestyle and personality:

Do you follow a regular, relaxed pattern in your life? If yes: add 1 point _/_

If you are older than retirement age, do you stay active in work or community affairs? If yes: add 1 point _7_

Are you good natured and placid? If yes: add 1 point _1_

Are you uptight, nervous, or tense? If yes: subtract 1 point _/_

If *happily* married: add 1 point _/_

Contributing longevity factors:

Do you get regular medical and dental checkups? If yes: add 1 point _/_

If you complain to your doctor about a minor ailment, does he give you a prescription immediately instead of telling you to adopt better health habits or to concentrate on good nutrition? If yes: subtract 1 point ___

Do you know for sure that your blood cholesterol is 190 to 170 or lower? If yes: add 1 point _/_

17

If your blood cholesterol is above 200: subtract 1
point ⎯

If your serum triglycerides are around 100 or
lower: add 1 point ⎯

If your serum triglycerides are above 120: subtract
2 points ⎯

Do you take any drugs on a long-term basis
without checking with your doctor from time to
time to see if this is still necessary? If yes: subtract
1 point ⎯

Alcohol consumption:

If you drink just an occasional beer or glass of
wine, or if you drink no alcohol at all: add 2 points *2*

If you drink strong liquor on a regular basis:
subtract 2 points ⎯

If you are a medium to heavy drinker: subtract 2
points ⎯

If you are a very heavy drinker (more than five
strong drinks per day): subtract another 2 points ⎯

Synergistic factors:

If ALL of the following apply: your weight is
normal, you don't smoke, you have a regular
exercise program, your nutrition habits are good:
add 2 points ⎯

If ALL of the following apply: you are at least 10
lbs. overweight, you smoke cigarettes, you have no
definite exercise program, you often eat quick
foods: subtract 3 points *-3* ⎯

You smoke cigarettes AND work in highly polluted
air: subtract 1 point ⎯

Special longevity factors:

If you receive nucleic acid therapy in combination
with blood analysis to make sure that uric acid
levels don't rise above normal: add 2 points   ___
If you ever received cell therapy or nucleic acid
injections: add 2 points   ___
If you receive(d) procaine therapy: add 2 points   ___
If you take organ-specific concentrates: add 2
points   ___

Add the following number of points, depending on your
age and sex:

Age:	man	woman
30 or under	41	42
31—40	39	40
41—50	37	39
51—60	35	37
61 and over	34	35

Your estimated life expectancy: ___

Included in these figures are causes of death due to accidents, shootings, killings, and a number of diseases. Eliminating these factors would increase life expectancies even further.

If your calculations indicate that you should have been dead
several years ago, this should ring a "red alert" in your head.
You are a bit like a gambler who has played Russian roulette
with a six-shooter more than six times and hasn't died yet.
You've been lucky, but the odds are against you.

Chapter 2

Taking the Mystery Out of Aging

Which species drinks the equivalent of four martinis per day, eats foods high in refined carbohydrates, and does no exercise?

The average businessman?

No—my laboratory mouse.

Aging is an extremely complex process. So far as we know today, about 40 separate factors can make us age at varying rates. As research continues, no doubt other aging and age-retarding factors will be discovered.

Extending life expectancies is often subdivided into three approaches: improving the quality of life (for example, by improving nutrition, doing the right exercises, lowering distress levels), preventing diseases, and interfering with the true causes of aging in order to go past the "maximum possible" lifespan. Each of these approaches has important ramifications that will be covered in Parts II, III, and IV of this book.

Since the average human lifespan is about 70 years and since the "maximum" human lifespan is at least 120, we are interested in all three areas. But this division of approaches to extending life expectancies is not, strictly speaking, correct. The three approaches overlap: For example, improving the quality of life can prevent some diseases. And as for the maximum possible lifespan, there is no real evidence it exists.

The Causes of Aging

Whether we are talking about extending "average" or "maximum" human lifespans, we must focus our attention on the cells in our body. The healthier all cells in our body are, the longer they will live and the better all organ systems will function.

Professor Leonard Hayflick of Stanford University has suggested that for every species there is a correlation between the maximum lifespan and the number of times a cell can reproduce itself by doubling. A few years ago he reported that certain human cells could double only a limited number of times, and this led him to conclude that there was a maximum human lifespan. Professor S. Gelfant, at the Miami Symposium on Theoretical Aspects of Aging, didn't quite agree. He reported that in cell cultures some cells stop dividing while others continue to do so, and that cells that had stopped dividing can be stimulated to divide again.

The "doublings-lifespan" theory raises some interesting questions. Is it possible to increase presently known cell doublings and thus extend the lifespan of cell cultures? If so, can this be done on human cells?

Lester Packer and James Smith, from the University of California, Berkeley, and the Veterans Administration Hospital, Martinez, showed that both these questions can be answered in one experiment. They treated human cells in culture with vitamin E and observed an increase of cell doublings from about 50 to more than 100. What is even more interesting is the fact that these cells didn't accumulate damage products and, in general, behaved like much younger cells. When they were subjected to ultraviolet light and high oxygen toxicity, the vitamin E also protected them against increased cell deaths.

I believe there is no final argument yet for either side of the lifespan controversy. But since both sides agree that the chemical reactions of aging can be interfered with, I predict there will be a time when human beings will live with healthy bodies for several hundred years or even longer.

A Practical Approach for Extending Lifespans

In our attempt to extend human lifespans, we won't worry whether we get results by interfering with true causes of aging or just by improving the functioning of specific cells in our body. It has now been proven that several different age-retarding factors acting together will have a stronger effect on the average lifespan than any single factor alone. These factors will also often be synergistic; this means that they enhance each other. If, for example, we find three separate factors that extend the average lifespan by 5 years each, we will often see an increase in lifespan of a little more than 15 years if the factors are applied together. That's why this book will stress the Multi-Factorial Approach as the most effective way for an individual to increase his or her life expectancy.

About 80 percent of all nonaccidental deaths in this country are caused by diseases of the arteries and lungs and by cancer. If we can improve the essential life factors, the incidence of these and disorders like hypoglycemia and diabetes will decrease strongly. Average life expectancies will increase sharply as more people get closer to the maximum human lifespan.

Increasing average lifespans and eliminating diseases will also give us enough time to search for true causes of aging and to break through the next barrier, the maximum lifespan. Our picture of this area is still somewhat vague. However, some key experiments performed on animals, including some done in my laboratory, suggest that we have to look at aging as a two-stage process. Various factors affect the entire body, but they also act specifically on the aging control center in the brain. This control center, also frequently called "the center of aging," appears to have a strong effect on the functioning of the various organ systems in the body. As we grow older, the control center doesn't send out the correct signals anymore and we feel the effects of aging.

The Aging Control Center in the Brain

A fascinating area in research recently opened up when it was demonstrated that the control center can be stimulated to send out the correct signals again. Formerly, it was believed that the cessation of hormone cycling in animals was due to the aging of the endocrine and sex organs: The glands just couldn't produce the hormones any more. However, when certain areas of the brain are stimulated mechanically, or when the synthesis of certain chemicals in the brain is improved, the control center can be made to send its "youth signals" again, and the glands again start producing hormones. It has been proven on animals that if the youth signals arrive correctly, the specific organs will function at their maximum possible capacity. In one of my own experiments, we succeeded in inducing these youth signals through the use of specific nutrients in combination with drugs that have no undesirable side effects.

23

A Corporate Comparison

If this appears complicated, let me compare the body to a large industrial company. The executives, the men and women who are the central organizers, can be compared to the control center in the brain. The overall functioning of the various departments, including the workers in them, in combination with the correct orders received from the executives, will then determine the output and efficiency of the entire company.

"Aging" of the company can now be compared to the executives getting lazy, not being up-to-date in their business, or one or more of them having problems (alcoholism, for example). The result is that they do not give the correct instructions for the best possible functioning of the firm. Naturally, aging also occurs in the different departments, where the supervisors spend too much time in the cafeteria, workers drink on the job, accidents happen, and machinery and equipment get worn out and are not repaired properly.

The overall rate of aging in the various departments can be prevented or slowed down by good maintenance and on-the-job training; these can be compared to good health habits. However, if the executives don't know what they are doing, and if special problems among them exist, this will ultimately lead to the ruin of the entire company.

Now, if we could come in with a "youth pill" and shape up the executive staff, make them act and perform like true, topnotch experts in their field giving the correct instructions, we would be well on the way toward making the company a true competitor in the business world. However, good instructions from the top won't do much good if the different departments, or possibly just one key department, are run down and not functioning as well as possible. What good are perfect instructions and smoothly functioning departments if the raw materials for making a product (in our case the nutrients) are incomplete or of a low quality?

This comparison shows just some of the reasons why it is so important to consider all the contributing factors to health and aging. (Interested professionals will find more technical details of my thinking explained in "The Combination Theory on Aging," published in the November 1976 issue of *American Laboratory.*)

The important points to keep in mind throughout this book are that anything that adversely affects our health will also cause an accelerated rate of aging, and that anything which can keep our cells functioning better will also help extend our life expectancy.

THE ANIMAL MODEL IN AGING RESEARCH

How can we verify that several factors acting together are more successful in extending our life expectancy than just one factor? Could we follow two groups of 1,000 people each for a lifetime? Could we limit them all to the same environment, while one group received all the compounds which have been shown to extend life expectancy and the others were under controlled conditions? Could we wait and see how long each group lived?

Perhaps we could study people in such a way over decades, but we can verify the Multi-Factorial Approach in much shorter lengths of time. There are other living beings with lifespans much shorter than ours and with organs very much like ours. Mice are classic examples. All their major organs are like ours. They are warm-blooded animals with the same basic cellular reactions as human beings. Rats, guinea pigs, monkeys, and other mammals are also physiologically similar to human beings and can be of tremendous help in studying our aging processes.

Normally, in studying aging in experiments, scientists begin with a number of animals divided into two groups. One group gets standard care, while the other receives some additional treatment that may extend lifespan. Experimentors then wait months, sometimes years, until the animals begin to die. Statistical data are collected and dead animals are dissected in search of any abnormalities. Then, after 50 percent of both groups have died, experimentors evaluate their findings and begin another experiment, varying the factors to improve upon their previous results.

If there is one factor to study, the major concern is to find the best possible results with the most reasonable quantities of that factor. If the effects of several factors are under study, the situation is far more complex, because optimal conditions may not be firmly established for all single factors. Furthermore, if we know the optimal conditions for some single factors, these may change when other factors are also involved. And even with short-lived animals, such as mice, one test takes at least 18 months.

As you may have guessed, I am a little impatient. In my experiments I have started to study the life extensions one can achieve by interfering with several aging factors at the same time.

Why don't I wait until the separate single factors are checked and evaluated in detail? For two major reasons. First of all, we have good indications that the single factors do have positive age-retarding effects. Second, if we were to wait until all the single factors were completely evaluated, we would probably be too old to make any use of the knowledge. I practice what I preach, and I would like to know if the things

I do have a positive or negative effect on my own lifespan and on health in general.

In our longevity studies and experiments on animals, about 700 animals were involved: rats, three different strains of mice, and guinea pigs. The results of these experiments, together with the most recent findings of other researchers, have until now been available only in professional circles. They will serve as the scientific basis for the material discussed and recommended in the chapters that follow.

We started with the hypothesis that by simultaneously blocking several of the internal processes that cause aging, we could achieve better life extensions. To verify this, we performed a series of longevity studies with mice.

A Laboratory Study

Group 1, the control group, received a standard treatment consisting of animal chow, tap water as the drinking fluid, and a normal-size environment. All in all, a typical, *average* group of mice.

Group 2 received our special attention and was exposed to a variety of life-extending factors; or, to be more precise, factors we believed to be life-extending. The environment was improved by adding hiding places, toys, and exercise wheels. Since animals also get lazy, they were exercised in a rotating drum twice per week. Vitamins, minerals, and compounds that affect the chemicals in the brain were added to their diet. Injections to revitalize the animals' cells were given at specific time intervals.

Group 3, which we called "the average businessmen," was subjected to several health insults. They received 20 percent refined sugar in their diet, were exposed to cigarette smoke regularly, and received the human equivalent of three strong alcoholic drinks per day. They did no exercise and their over-all health habits were very bad.

As the experiment progressed, great differences in average lifespans were observed. Group 3 had a lifespan about 30 percent shorter than Group 1, mainly due to an increase in cancer of the various organ systems. Group 2 showed an increase in average lifespans of about 100 percent over Group 3, due mainly to a strong decrease in cancer. Animals in Group 2 also looked younger, lost their hair later than the "mistreated" animals, and were more active in general.

"Average" Lifespans

Group 3		
	Group 1	
		Group 2

The emphasis in these studies was on superb nutrition and good health habits, two factors that are available to everybody and that show the lowest possible risk of having negative side effects.

THE COMBINATION THEORY ON AGING

These experiments prove that the Multi-Factorial Approach is valid. We *can* interfere with aging by blocking several aging processes simultaneously. The results also show that the genetic factor, which is often blamed for the aging process, is not the sole determinant when it comes to average, and even "maximum," lifespans.

We are often told that what applies to animals doesn't have to apply to humans; this is true to a degree. But in the field of health, animal experiments have often shown the way. In addition, there is already some proof that several contributing factors work together to improve health and longevity in humans.

A Longevity Study

In July of 1974, a team at UCLA studied a population of 7,000 people and found that good habits of daily life are definitely related to health in general and longevity in particular.

The researchers studied specific habits ranging from sleep to smoking cigarettes, routine of meal intake, weight, and others. When the survey was evaluated, it was found that the various habits were cumulative.

Sleep: Men who slept between seven and eight hours a night had a lower mortality rate than men who slept more or less. The best amount of sleep for women was seven hours or a little less.

Smoking: The least risk of death was experienced by those who never smoked. Mortality risk was highest for those who smoked two or more packs of cigarettes per day.

Drinking: People who never drank alcoholic beverages had about the same mortality as people who drank moderately. The highest risk was observed for heavy drinkers (those who had five or more drinks per day).

Exercise: This factor was extremely important. Those who exercised regularly had a mortality rate only about half as high as those who never exercised.

Eating habits: The erratic eater had much worse health than the person who ate three regular meals. Breakfast was found to be of particular value.

29

Weight: A few percentage points over the optimum weight didn't play an important role, but as soon as 20 percent was reached, the death rate went up.

The people who were surveyed were rated from 1 to 7, according to the number of health habits they practiced. For men at age 45 who scored 0 to 3, the average life expectancy was an additional 21.6 years. However, if they did relatively well in six or seven health practices, their additional life expectancy was 33.1 years, an improvement of almost 12 years. The extensions would have been even more dramatic if these people had been able to use some of the additional life extending factors we are now working with.

From these findings you can see that our animal model holds up pretty well. Humans who do almost everything wrong have an approximate average lifespan of 60 years, yet the presently established maximum is at least 110 to 120 years. The average lifespan of animals who do everything wrong is about half that of animals who do everything right and get the life-extending treatment. This is a superb agreement of an experimental animal model with the actual human "average" and "maximum" lifespans. In addition, there are already indications that we can go past this established "maximum."

THE REVERSAL OF AGING

Scientists in Madison, Wisconsin, are well on their way toward developing a technique that will actually reverse the aging process. Dr. Johan Bjorksten and his associates at Bjorksten Research Laboratories have focused their attention on "cross-linkers," chemicals that can hook together the large molecules within our cells. When this occurs, the cross-linked molecules can no longer do their jobs correctly and instead interfere with normal cell functions. This bonding process is about as useful as handcuffing together all the employees of a large factory: Under such a handicap, they are hardly in a position to do their jobs. As cross-linking advances in cells, so does aging. But Dr. Bjorksten has found an enzyme that can break the disabling bonds between cross-linked molecules. Preliminary tests on mice show the enzyme can increase life expectancies without harmful side effects, and as further studies are carried out its safety and effectiveness for human beings will be assessed.

Evaluating the Latest Findings

Good research results reported in reputable scientific journals are the most reliable data one can find. These include long-term research done on animals, which can sometimes be more conclusive than short-term experiments on humans. Although some of these research results are not yet 100 percent proved, I am willing to accept them as long as there is no danger in their applications. By evaluating these results, we can come up with good advice for a large proportion of the healthy population.

It is possible that the general rules for prolonging life in healthy people may not be advisable for certain others. Individual biochemistries are so different that it is just impossible to prescribe one set of rules for everyone. Even though we are now convinced, for example, that large doses of vitamin C are very beneficial to the majority, it is possible that a few may be adversely affected.

The question we have to answer about life-prolonging treatments is one of balancing good effects against bad ones. If 97 out of 100 people are affected in a positive way while 3

31

are affected in a negative way, which is more important: the improvement in health of the 97 or the bad effects on the 3? This kind of situation is not unusual. In many areas of medicine, treatments good for one person might not be good for another.

Personally, I would take the 97 percent chance of improving my health or prolonging my life without worrying about the 3 percent chance of adverse effects.

Where your health is concerned, you must make your own decisions. If you know of any condition or injury that would cause you to limit your participation in a program that would be beneficial to others, then by all means work within your limitations. And if you don't know your limitations, maybe this is the time to have that checkup you've been putting off for so long.

Before you begin any new health regimen, remember: It's your body and only you can take care of it. Take time now to get to know yourself as only you can.

Part II

Improving the Quality of Life

The United States Public Health Service recognizes only 3 million of our population of 210 million—about 1½ percent—as being healthy.

Chapter 3

The Ideal Nutrition

In Helsinki, health officials have warned Finns that sugar is so dangerous they would ban it as a food additive if it were newly discovered.

The average American consumes over 100 pounds of sugar per year.

1983406

THE NUTRITION QUIZ   Yes No

1. Do you prefer fresh foods to canned and so-called "fast foods"?   — —
2. Do you use nonfat milk rather than cream in your coffee or tea; do you minimize your use of butter as well as margarine; and do you cut the fat off your steak?   — —
3. Do you make an effort to limit your intake of refined carbohydrate foods like sugar, white flour, processed cereals, and even honey?   — —
4. Does your normal diet contain sufficient roughage (lots of vegetables, whole fruits

      instead of fruit juices, whole grain
      products)?   — —

5. Do you realize that you need a limited
      amount of polyunsaturates (approximately
      two to three teaspoons per day) in your
      diet?   — —

6. Do you know for sure that your blood
      cholesterol level is around 190 to 170 or
      lower and your triglyceride level 100 or
      lower?   — —

7. Is your diet extremely high in proteins?   — —

8. Are you over-weight?   — —

9. Do you consume more than one can of cola
      or other sugar-containing soft drink or diet
      soda per day?   — —

If you answered "yes" to 1 through 6 and "no" to 7 through 9, you could skim this chapter and then move on to the next.

If your answer to 6 was "yes," answering 2 correctly will be less important; if only 6 was answered with a "no," have your cholesterol and triglyceride levels checked by a doctor as soon as possible.

A Case History

I was once consulted by a 36-year-old woman who reported that both she and her husband, 38, felt much older than their age, got tired easily, and had little zest for life. Both were under the impression they followed good health habits; they purchased high quality foods and took supplements of vitamins A and C. They had consulted their family doctor, who had found nothing basically wrong with them.

First I asked them each to get a blood analysis. When they

did, it showed that their blood cholesterol and triglyceride levels were too high, and certain other factors were not in the correct ranges. The amounts of cholesterol and fats in the blood, expressed as cholesterol and triglyceride (chemical name for fat) levels, are believed to be coronary heart disease risk factors (more about this in Chapter 11). The results of the blood analysis were not surprising, because they were both overweight and consumed a high percentage—nearly half—of their daily caloric intake in the form of animal fat.

These people informed me they were getting regular exercise but I discovered that they, like most people, just didn't do enough of it. Their exercise level expressed in calories burnt up was less than 1,000 per week, when it should have been at least 3,000.

In addition, questioning their eating habits revealed a strong possibility that their calcium-to-phosphorus ratios, important for normal functioning of the thyroid gland, were out of balance and their fiber intake was relatively low.

To improve their overall health, I gave these people the appropriate dietary recommendations to lower their fat intake (which also brought the proportion of fibers up), balance their vitamin intake, and normalize their calcium-to-phosphorus ratio.

After about two weeks on the new program they noticed improvements. Then they also increased their exercise level by walking longer distances at an accelerated pace, and soon they felt much better than before.

Many people, like those described in this case history, are under the impression they are following sound health habits when, under professional scrutiny, it can be discovered that they are following paths that can lead to serious problems. Even doctors and other health specialists often have mistaken ideas about nutrition.

The Need for Better Nutrition

The importance of good nutrition was recently demonstrated in two of my studies, among others. In one survey of flight attendants, which would almost place stewardesses on the "endangered species" list, we examined nutritional habits relating to protein, fats, polyunsaturates, fibers, vitamins, and calcium, and found that only about 15 percent fulfilled our suggested requirements. In another experiment we studied the effect of improved nutrition on the average lifespans of test animals. In the exercise-nutrition-longevity study on mice, the treated animals achieved an average extension of 35 percent beyond the average lifespan of the control group. They also looked younger and were more active.

The Ideal Diet

Food consumption in the main consists of fats, carbohydrates, and proteins. Fats, including oils, should be part of the diet, but a small part for most people. The proportion of complex carbohydrates like vegetables, bran, and whole-grain products should be high, and consumption of refined carbohydrates like sugar and foods made from refined flour should be kept low. Protein intake should be rather on the high side; we'll see later how to calculate all your nutritional needs.

Naturally, due to our biochemical individuality, there will be some exceptions to these rules. For example, there are people who have a very high rate of metabolism and who burn up foods very fast. For such persons, as long as blood cholesterol and triglyceride levels are low, the percentage of calories from fat could be far above what it should be for another person. And, as we'll see, anyone with abnormal blood sugar levels will have to take special dietary precautions.

Food Shopping for Supernutrition

Nutrition is a complicated subject on which even the experts don't always agree. Nevertheless, it's easy to follow some basic rules about food selection in order to try to get what's best for you.

1. Read the label. Does it sound like the inventory of a chemical company? Don't buy it! Be especially wary of artificial food coloring, sodium nitrite, and sodium nitrate.

2. Emphasize high-quality foods like fresh vegetables, fruits, whole grain products, and fresh seafood. Try to avoid canned and processed foods.

3. Don't buy food items high in sugar, refined carbohydrates, or fats and oils.

4. Buy lots of food items that are high in fibers. Some good examples are carrots, celery, broccoli, and other vegetables, as well as whole grain and bran products. Select whole fruits over fruit juices.

5. Buy a variety of different protein foods like lowfat dairy products, lean meats, fish, nuts, beans, and other vegetable proteins. Don't eat just one type of protein.

6. Buy at least part of your food in a reliable health-food store to reduce your overall intake of additives and leftover pesticides.

The Dangers of Pesticides

Years ago, I was employed by a chemical company as a pesticides researcher. The firm could have explored many alternative means of controlling insects and other pests, but the corporate leadership always abandoned them when it became clear they would generate no new patents, or when the anticipated profit margin was low. We really can't blame industry for acting this way. In a capitalistic system investors are not expected to put their money into projects having anticipated returns below the projected development expenses. Government grants and university research theoretically should fill this gap, but all too often they don't. Therefore, it is up to each of us to do what we can to limit our intake of harmful chemicals.

Traces of pesticides remain on foods consumed by everyone. Since the latest available information indicates that the average American now ingests more than five pounds of additives per year, it is especially important to limit any additional intake of chemicals, especially pesticides. We know for sure that some of them can increase the risk of cancer and other diseases.

In a Senate hearing in April 1976, 12 present and former Environmental Protection Agency (EPA) scientists testified that adequate evidence for the safety of commonly used pesticides was not available. A cancer specialist, among others, testified that data supplied by the pesticides industry about the safety of its products were, in several cases, "misleading and distorted." Of 25 industry reports on 23 such pesticides, only 1 was satisfactory; the rest he described as "uniformly bad."

In other reports we read that atrazine (a weed killer) can cause cancer, and that pronamide (a compound used to keep the turf on golf courses trim) is being investigated by the EPA as a possible cancer hazard.

Washing fruits and vegetables with regular liquid soap, but not with a detergent, and buying organic produce should decrease our pesticide intake to a level that our body can handle. Dr. Hans Nieper from Germany reported to the International Academy of Preventive Medicine in 1977 that detergents are highly suspect as a major cause of fat accumulation in the liver. Soap and organic cleaners, bought in your health food store, can reduce this risk.

The Food Industry Disaster

Unfortunately the business ethic also dictates that the motivation of the food industry is profit rather than nutrition. Even though very small quantities of the following foods, when consumed only occasionally, probably have little effect on the health of most of us, eating them regularly would be an invitation to trouble.

Canned foods: With fewer vitamins, more additives, and an undesirable mineral balance, canned foods provide a decidedly lower nutritional value than fresh.

Processed meats: Additives like sodium nitrite and nitrate are established cancer hazards. In addition, bacon, ham and other processed meats expose us to hormone leftovers from animal feeding.

Sugar: Medical researchers are connecting more and more diseases with our high sugar intake, and a Senate committee is considering urging Americans to cut their sugar consumption by 40 percent. Even so, food manufacturers are adding sugar to more and more products, including hot dogs, salad dressings, and cold cuts. These companies pay only about nine cents a pound for sugar, making it one of the cheapest and therefore most profitable ingredients available.

Processed cereals: Commercial processing not only removes up to 90 percent of the nutritional value of whole grains; it also increases the amount of sugar we eat. Many cereals contain as much as 50 percent sugar, though you sometimes can't

41

tell by reading the list of ingredients. Cereal producers often use a variety of relatively cheap sugar-based ingredients, such as malt syrup, corn syrup, and brown sugar, listing each separately. Since the package might show "wheat bran" and "rolled oats" first, a cereal-buyer might think these are the major ingredients, even though the product consists mostly of sugar.

Homogenized milk: According to heart specialists, homogenized milk serves as a carrier for xanthine oxidase, an enzyme that can damage arteries. The high fat content, if not burned up by a person, is another coronary heart disease (CHD) risk factor. (More about this in Chapter 11.)

Frozen dinners: These are yet another example of how mother nature's products can be mistreated, devalued, pumped full of additives, and then sold as convenience foods.

Breads and other products made from refined flour: In the process of making refined flour from wheat, up to 80 percent of 24 major nutrients is\removed. Then four ingredients are added to the remaining material and it is sold to you as "enriched." A key factor here is the lack of fiber.

Juices: Have you ever counted the pure juices available in your grocery store? Most products in the juice section are called "drink," "punch," or "cocktail" because they are not juices. They contain mainly water and artificial flavors with only a very small percentage of real juice, and that little part is often reconstituted from concentrates using tap water.

This was only a short supermarket review from the gerontologist's point of view. A detailed analysis by Max Huberman, President of the National Nutritional Foods Association, appeared in the April, May, and June 1977 issues of *Let's Live* magazine. I strongly recommend it to interested readers.

OUR CHILDREN

The most innocent victims of the food industry disaster are our children. Advertising is hitting them hard with insinuations that sugar-rich junk foods are nutritious. We reward children for being good by giving them candy. The foods commonly sold in school cafeterias are of the lowest nutritional value.

"Junk foods create learning and behavioral problems. Symptoms like aggressive criminal-type behavior, inability to read well, poor concentration, falling asleep in school, and hyperactivity are very often traceable to foods," says Dr. William Philpott, an Oklahoma City psychiatrist.

In 1975, the Montreal Island, Canada, school system banned the sale of junk foods in all 525 member schools. "And today our children are more attentive and less restless. There are less fights and trouble," William Neuheimer, principal of St. Gabriel's Grammar School in Montreal, said in 1977.

Food Preparation for Supernutrition

The importance of supernutrition in the overall anti-aging, health-promoting program can't be overemphasized. Many excellent books have been devoted to this subject alone. I often recommend *Supernutrition for Healthy Hearts* by Richard Passwater, Ph.D. (Dial Press), and *Psychodietetics* by E. Cheraskin, M.D. (Stein and Day), for those who consult me.

Readers interested in following a supernutrition diet should find these guidelines for food preparation useful:

1. If you cook for yourself, high-quality fresh foods will cost you no more (and perhaps less) than the so-called conve-

nience foods. Home economists have estimated that two people can eat well and wisely for about $3.50 to $4.50 per day.

2. Serve a glass of quality spring water, or carbon-filtered water, with every meal.

3. When cooking vegetables try to leave them whole and unpeeled. Just clean them with a brush and possibly with an organic cleanser, but not with a detergent.

4. Cook vegetables as little as possible, keeping them slightly crisp. Use a pressure cooker.

5. When you get the urge for a snack, try munching raw vegetables, raw nuts, high protein chips, lowfat yogurt, etc.

6. Use a vegetable shredder to make delicious multivegetable salads and soups.

7. Get yourself a sprouter and a supply of various seeds. Use sprouts in salads, on sandwiches, or as in-between snacks.

8. Prepare meats and fish as soon as possible after buying them. Avoid excessive amounts of fat, butter, or oils in the preparation of these and other foods.

9. Beverages like tea or coffee should be used in moderation. Don't make them very strong and serve them only when somebody asks for them.

10. For pleasing drinks between or with meals use herb tea (which lacks caffeine) or vegetable bouillon from your health-food store.

11. Always prepare a cross-section of different types of foods and serve at least some of them raw.

What About Fasting?

Good results have been claimed for fasting, but biochemistry suggests that health improvements were achieved only because people were not allowed their usual bad nutritional habits during the fast. Such benefits could have been achieved with milder, less risky methods. Fasting, the intake of nothing but water, can, over an extended period, expose the body to serious dangers. I do not recommend it for most people. I would especially discourage anyone with diabetes or some other chronic disease from fasting. The water-soluble vitamins, minerals, and proteins are not stored by our bodies, and to deprive ourselves of these important compounds is potentially very serious. During a fast the glucose level must be maintained, and under such strict conditions this is only possible by the conversion of lean muscle tissue; this too is undesirable. Nutrients for perfect functioning of our nervous system are not supplied while fasting, and depression on a short-term basis and earlier senility on a long-term basis are definite risks.

How Much? How Many?

So far we have discussed in general terms the basic rules that can get you started on a reasonably balanced diet. However, for the best possible results, more precise calculations are needed. The rest of this chapter will present the quantitative side of nutrition.

I believe that the quantitative approach is very important for understanding nutrition and that it provides some of the easiest means available to us for interfering with the aging process. But there's no denying that it's complicated. If it seems too tedious or too difficult for you, ask your doctor about the *Nutrition, Health, and Activity Profile*, an educational questionnaire that can analyze your health habits, including the nutritional value of your diet, by computer; or send a self-addressed envelope to P. O. Box 5252, Torrance, Ca. 90510 and ask for details. For those interested in calculating their own nutritional needs, here are some guidelines.

Proteins: A cross-section of proteins will provide the best possible supply of amino acids, chemicals your body uses to manufacture many essential substances. If a major proportion of protein comes from plant sources, as in a vegetarian diet, a possible methionine (sulfur amino acid) deficiency can occur and absorption of the protein will be slightly reduced.

The most widely accepted protein recommendations are those made by the FAO/WHO (World Health Organization) of 1973. Taking into account numerous factors ranging from nitrogen requirements to the digestibility and quality of proteins, this committee came up with a recommendation of 0.57 grams of egg protein per kilogram (2.2 pounds) of body weight per day as a desirable level for 97.5 percent of the population. (Egg protein is used as a standard because it is nutritionally similar to a combination of other common proteins.) According to this, a 150-pound person would need only about 38 grams of protein per day. For purposes of comparison, there are about 8 grams of protein in one glass of milk, 6 grams in one egg, and 21 grams in 3 ounces of fish or beef.

On a national level, numerous countries now recommend 1 gram of protein per kilogram of body weight per day; this number takes into account a slight safety margin.

In a 1976 study, Dr. Nevin Scrimshaw of MIT concluded that the FAO's proposed protein standard of 0.57 grams per kilogram was incorrect. Half the test subjects receiving such a diet lost lean muscle mass, an undesirable form of weight loss and a sign that the metabolic system was functioning abnormally. Scrimshaw found that the body's protein needs should be computed not from weight, but from daily calorie expenditure. His studies show that for every calorie used in a day, the body, regardless of age, needs to consume .11 grams of "body protein." Since the body manufactures this type of protein itself—using a gram of protein from food to

46

produce 4 to 5 grams of "body protein," according to Scrimshaw—we can easily compute how much protein a person should include in his daily diet.

After adding a small percentage to ensure against any deficiency, we come up with this formula for the daily protein requirement:

$$0.03 \times \text{daily caloric expenditure} = \text{protein requirement in grams per day.}$$

How to calculate your daily caloric expenditure: Keep track of all the food, including drinks, you consume in one typical day. Then add up the caloric contents of all these foods with the help of a calorie counter (sold in most bookstores at modest cost). The result is your daily caloric intake, and if you neither gain nor lose weight, it is also your daily caloric expenditure.

For example, a man whose daily caloric expenditure is about 2,500 calories would calculate his protein needs as follows:

$$0.03 \times 2,500 = 75 \text{ grams per day.}$$

Critics of the high-protein diet often argue that countries in which the protein intake is high also have higher rates of cancer. However, if one examines the eating patterns of people in such countries, one will also find that their fiber and roughage intake is very low. Professor Denis Burkitt in Australia has demonstrated that fiber can prevent colon-rectal cancer and other cancers of the digestive tract. A low-fiber diet is also associated with a low intake of antioxidants like vitamins C and E; several research papers have emphasized the importance of antioxidants in cancer prevention.

In support of higher protein intake levels are longevity studies on animals as well as some recent work on humans by

E. Cheraskin, M.D., chairman of the department of oral medicine at Alabama University. Dr. Cheraskin determined that human tryptophane (an essential amino acid) needs are somewhere in the range of 1,100 to 1,800 mg per day. Since we know the tryptophane content of proteins, we can now translate this number into actual protein requirements, and this suggests an intake of at least 90 to 150 grams per day.

Fat: The average American diet derives about 40 percent of its calories from fat. This, according to the experts in the field of heart disease, is too high; some like to see it at about 34 percent while others recommend levels as low as 10 percent. A range of 20 to 34 percent appears reasonable.

To determine the percentage of your total caloric intake you receive from fat, add up the number of grams of fat you consume in your foods per day. So many widely available books on nutrition contain tables of food contents that I have not included them here. Refer to them to find out the number of grams of fat in the foods you consumed during a typical day. Now multiply this number by nine (one gram of fat yields 9 calories), and then calculate the percentage of these calories in your daily caloric expenditure (which is the same as your daily caloric intake if your weight doesn't change).

For example, if a man has a daily caloric intake of about 2,500 calories, and the number of grams of fat in the food consumed in an average day add up to 140, he is consuming 140 times 9, or 1,260 calories from fat. Dividing 1,260 by 2,500 we get .504, or 50.4 percent; far too high. In order to get below 34 percent, this man should reduce his fat intake to below 94 grams per day (34 percent of 2,500 is 850 calories; 850 divided by 9 gives 94).

Since the major problem associated with a high percentage of calories from fat is a high triglyceride level, one could just have the triglycerides checked by a doctor, and then reduce fat and increase exercise more and more until the triglycerides drop to a normal level. Your prevention-oriented doctor knows the details for such an approach.

Fibers: Fibers move foods faster through the digestive tract, thus preventing the formation of carcinogens. Fibers also help to control serum cholesterol levels, an important indicator of heart disease. If you eat a lot of junk foods, chances are that you are fiber deficient.

Exact norms for fiber intake have not yet been established but a minimum intake of about 5 grams appears reasonable for a 150-pound person; add or subtract 1 gram if you weigh more or less. Tables of food contents usually also list the fiber content of foods.

Calcium and Phosphorus: A NASA study recently showed that we need about 1,000 to 1,500 mg of calcium per day and that the ratio of calcium to phosphorus in our foods should be about 1:1 but not more than 1:2. According to a 1957 study, the calcium intake for the average person was only about 400 mg per day, and the calcium-to-phosphorus ratio was about 1:2.5. In the meantime, the consumption of milk (a major source of calcium) has gone down, and the consumption of cola (which contains lots of phosphorus but no calcium) has gone up, changing the calcium-to-phosphorus ratio even more. In animals, a diet high in phosphorus and low in calcium has been shown to induce secondary hyperparathyroidism, which is associated with a loss of calcium, demineralization of bone, and muscle pains.

Only precise calculations of the calcium and phosphorus contents of your foods through the use of tables of food contents can show you where you stand in this critical area. It isn't safe to increase your calcium consumption without establishing an exact need for it, because an excess of calcium can lead to other disorders (although a slight excess is usually tolerated without difficulties, especially if a person is on a high-protein diet).

The present recommended daily allowance of calcium is 800 mg. Exact calculations of your intake of calcium, and also of the other minerals, make the use of a computer a necessity.

Carbohydrates: These are subdivided into refined and complex carbohydrates.

Refined carbohydrates include sugar, refined cereals, and foods made from white flour. The breakdown of these foods into glucose in the digestive tract is very fast and results in an upsurge of blood sugar. In a healthy person this rise in the glucose level stimulates the insulin mechanism and the glucose level is brought down to normal. However, if we constantly subject ourselves to changes in the glucose level through intake of refined carbohydrates, the insulin mechanism becomes very sensitive and overreacts; the result is low blood sugar, hypoglycemia.

Complex carbohydrates (vegetables, bran and whole grain products, fruits with a low sugar content) are broken down more slowly and release glucose into the blood stream over a much longer period of time. Thus, if all the other factors (exercise, metabolism rate, etc.) are right, it is possible to keep the blood sugar within a certain correct range without aggravating the insulin mechanism.

Evaluating all these nutritional factors and putting them into precise perspective can be very difficult and time consuming; that's why I recommend the use of computerized nutrition evaluations. However, the principles outlined earlier in this chapter will put you on the right track.

Chapter 4

Exercise for Life

The men of the Tarahoe Indian tribe, in competitions, run 100 miles per day for five days, kicking a wooden ball; the women run only 60 miles per day.

In the prevention of heart disease good results are being achieved by people who merely go for an extended walk twice per day.

How much exercise are you doing?

	The Exercise Quiz	Yes	No
1.	Do you have a regular exercise program?	—	—
2.	Does it combine endurance exercises with muscle and flexibility exercises?	—	—
3.	Do you warm up before doing your exercises?	—	—
4.	Are you overweight?	—	—
5.	Do you exercise even when you have a		

cold, respiratory ailment, or other
temporary illness? — —

6. Do you use rubber suits or belts and/or
   extended time periods in the whirlpool,
   steam room, or sauna to lose weight? — —

7. Do you do exercise against the wishes of
   your doctor? — —

8. Do you often try to "squeeze in" a quick
   hour of exercise during a stressful day
   when you are already tired? — —

9. If you're over 35, or if you are out of
   shape and haven't exercised in a long time,
   do you think it is necessary to consult your
   doctor before you start your exercise
   program? — —

10. If you can't do exercises, do you take
    physical therapy, massages, etc.? — —

In order to pass this quiz you should have answered "yes"
to questions 1, 2, 3, 9, and 10; "no" to questions 4, 5, 6, 7,
and 8.

The most important questions are 1, 2, 4, 9, and 10. If you
answered these correctly, but made mistakes in some others,
you could move on to the next chapter but make sure to come
back to this chapter later.

The link between exercise and lifespan was established as
long as fifty years ago when papers in the German medical
literature demonstrated that physical activity improved overall health, reduced susceptibility to many diseases, and extended best possible functioning of the various organ systems. In experiments on animals, exercise was found to
increase average lifespans by up to 40 percent. It is all too
easy to find excuses for avoiding exercise: weather conditions,

pressing schedules, and lack of equipment are some of the more common ones. But men and women who exercise regularly not only test out as healthier by a variety of standards, they feel better and have more energy for life in general.

Exercise to Prevent Illness

Years ago studies demonstrated the connection between exercise and the prevention of heart disease; today most people are aware of the correlation. More recently, research findings also demonstrated that exercise can be an important factor in cancer prevention, and supporting evidence is accumulating at a steady rate. Only a few months ago here in the United States, the relationship of hypoglycemia and diabetes to lack of exercise was confirmed by experiments on humans.

The role of exercise in maintaining a healthy blood sugar level may be explained by the facts that exercise stimulates muscle buildup, and that an increase in muscle mass is directly related to a higher base metabolism. It's not only that people who exercise burn up more calories. Even without exercising, a person with a larger muscle mass will have a higher metabolism rate and therefore will be able to handle a high-calorie insult to his body without gaining weight.

In diseases like hypoglycemia and diabetes, the problem lies in the limited capacity of the body to handle glucose, a form of sugar. This situation is worsened by the presence of large amounts of fat in the blood, the triglycerides. When we eat carbohydrates, they wind up as glucose in the blood. This sugar is stored in the liver and muscle tissue as glycogen and is released back into the blood when glucose levels drop.

The initial impact of glucose on the body is strongest when we eat refined carbohydrates and sugar. If we eat complex carbohydrates, the glucose is released much more slowly into the blood stream, and blood sugar levels don't jump so high because we are burning it up at the same time. Anybody with a well exercised body and/or a larger muscle mass will be able to handle a larger amount of glucose because the muscle also serves as a buffer by converting glucose into glycogen.

At the Veterans Administration Hospital in Lexington, Kentucky, Dr. James Anderson demonstrated that diabetics with blood sugar counts as high as 350 (just below 100 is normal) were freed from their dependence on drugs with an exercise program that featured, among other things, walking for half an hour directly after every meal. A diet high in complex carbohydrates and roughage, low in fats, supported this preventive approach.

It is often hard to convince women to do exercises because they are worried that they might develop a muscular body. On the contrary, lean muscle tissue gives a woman the firm, round shape which men find so attractive; lack of it causes cellulite. We are not asking women to do 300-pound bench presses, but some kind of exercise with the equipment in the gymnasium is definitely advisable to maintain a normal amount of lean muscle tissue and to keep it functioning well.

Even though there are many ways you can exercise, outdoors and indoors, for a large percentage of people these possibilities are minimized due to their environment and climate. Exercising in the winter on a regular basis is easier for a person who lives on the beach in California than for someone who lives in New York City. Buying your own exercise equipment is expensive, and doing exercises by yourself in your own home just isn't too exciting. For these, and other reasons, people are joining health clubs in increasing numbers.

How to Chose Your Health Club

If you decide to join a health club, there are a few simple questions you should ask before you sign.

1. Does it have trained instructors and nutrition information?

2. Does it have branches or affiliates in other cities? If you move, you don't want to start all over again, especially if joining requires an initiation fee.

3. Do its hours of operation fit your work schedule?

4. Besides the basic exercise equipment, does it have other sports facilities like tennis courts, golf, sailing?

5. Does it have a masseur or masseuse?

6. Do you get at least part of your money back if you decide that you don't want to continue with this club?

How to Start Your Exercise Program

Too often, in launching a physical fitness regimen, people try to do things too fast. The result is that they overdo things and thus induce medical problems.

Start slowly, build up, and give your body some rest between exercises. Do exercises in combination with a concerted health approach. Start with walking, then walk longer distances; then walk longer distances at accelerated speeds; then add some jogging. If you are a member of a health club, listen to your instructor and join one of the exercise classes taught by him or her.

DO'S AND DON'TS OF EXERCISE

The advisory board of the Chicago Health Clubs and the Tennis Corporation of America, which includes leading specialists in the areas of health and physical recreation, has worked out a list of do's and don'ts that summarizes the most basic rules for a good exercise program.

Follow these directions. The right exercise program will help you to improve your energy, endurance, and resistance to diseases, while extending your life expectancy. Exercise is also a key factor in losing weight, maintaining cardiovascular fitness, and preventing the formation of cellulite.

Training Tips From the Advisory Board

Health and Tennis Corporation of America*

Preface: Exercise can and should be enjoyable! Exercise is a natural and safe way to improve health, promote physical fitness and enhance the enjoyment of life. Exercise can help to improve appearance, help reduce excess fat and help to improve abilities in recreational activities and athletic participation.

The following training tips will insure that you get the most out of your exercise program in a safe and effective way. These principles are applicable to normal healthy individuals of both sexes at all ages.

DO's

    1. DO make exercise a regular habit. Set aside a specific

*I am grateful to the Chicago Health Clubs and the Tennis Corporation of America for letting me use this material

time during the day as you would for eating and sleeping.

2. DO warm up! Begin each exercise session with 5 to 15
   minutes of light exercises preparing *all* muscles, ten-
   dons, and joints for increasingly more vigorous activity.

3. DO "cool down" actively during the last 5 minutes of
   each exercise session, using exercises which will help
   to relax all muscles.

4. DO balance your exercise program by including and
   mixing: endurance-type exercises such as walking, jogging, running, cycling, and swimming; exercises to
   build up adequate muscle strength; flexibility exercises; and exercises to improve motor skills.

5. DO a minimum of three strength and muscle endurance workouts per week. Cardio-Vascular-Respiratory
   endurance exercises should be performed daily.

6. DO elevate your pulse rate into the range of 130–160
   beats per minute when performing endurance exercise.

7. DO keep a daily record of your attendance and exercise
   efforts and a weekly record of your weight and of any
   problems encountered.

8. DO periodically evaluate the progress of your physical
   fitness exercise program.

9. DO, if over 35 years of age, consult with your physician
   for a physical examination and, most desirable, for a
   Functional Capacity Test prior to participating in any
   physical fitness program.

10. DO combine dietary and exercise routines to help
    maintain a desirable body weight (without excess
    fat).

11. DO a strength and muscle endurance exercise pro-
    gram that works every major muscle group. It is not

wise to use only selected exercises. This can lead to a muscular strength imbalance.

DON'Ts

1. *DON'T* perform any exercise program against the wishes of your physician.
2. *DON'T* exercise vigorously within one hour after any major meal.
3. *DON'T* exercise if you have a common cold, respiratory ailment, specific or unspecific infection, or any other illness or physical handicap—without medical approval.
4. *DON'T* strain to perform an exercise. Increase the intensity of exercise only when it becomes easy.
5. *DON'T* sit or lie down immediately after exercising. Keep moving (at least 10 minutes) to facilitate recovery from your previous efforts.
6. *DON'T* use rubber suits, rubber belts, whirlpool, steam, and sauna baths as a means of attempting to lose weight. These devices merely dehydrate the body and do not burn up the excess body fat.
7. *DON'T* abuse your body with excesses of food, alcohol, and nicotine.
8. *DON'T* go on a "fad" diet. A calorically balanced diet, which includes the four basic food groups, is the only sensible and correct approach to diet and nutrition management.
9. *DON'T* try to reduce more than two pounds per week.
10. *DON'T* use passive exercise equipment such as rollers or vibrators. These devices are not effective for eliminating fat or increasing muscle tone and can be dangerous when used as massaging agents.
11. *DON'T* routinely exercise to the extent of physical dis-

comfort and real pain—but enjoy your physical experiences.

REMEMBER

A sedentary person will begin to feel better after a few workouts. However, it will take a longer time to observe physical and physiological improvements.

Soreness, associated with exercises that are newly performed, may be minimized by starting at lower intensity levels. Progressive adjustment of exercise intensity assures comfortable and continued improvement. Training must be *progressive, regular, frequent,* and sufficiently *vigorous.*

Each individual has a different exercise tolerance. Train within your own tolerance.

The cumulative physiological changes induced by exercise are the very best and most effective means for achieving permanent fat reduction and normalization of body weight. Lack of exercise causes premature physiological aging and deterioration of functional capacity. For best results, exercise must be combined with other good health habits.

Rules for Rest

Just as you should follow certain guidelines in exercising your body, so should you follow a few pointers in how you rest your body.

Statistical data suggest that seven to eight hours of sleep is best for the majority of people. During the rest period the body reaches a state of equilibrium once metabolic leftovers have been moved out of the cells and into the urine. Repair and regeneration occur when the body can devote less effort to other functions. Finally, when a normal state of equilibrium has been achieved, the body wakes up. The process of reaching this normal equilibrium will take a little longer after a mentally and physically active day. But if a person consistently sleeps longer than seven to eight hours, this is a sign that health habits and nutrition need improvement.

In any case, you should try to sleep in a cool room. Your body temperature decreases slightly during a period of rest, and your metabolism rate reaches a low. Excretion of oxidation products is best under such conditions. Sleeping in a cool room lowers the metabolism even more, and a normal equilibrium can be achieved faster; that means one will need less sleep. Sleeping in an overheated room increases the metabolism rate, and the time required to achieve equilibrium will be longer; you might even wake up tired. Living and working in overheated rooms has the same effect. So, turning down the thermostat doesn't only save energy, it can also extend your lifespan.

Weight Loss Through Exercise

Many books on how to lose weight appear to have little respect for your health and are, in their faddist approach, often outright dangerous. Diets like "protein and lots of water only," and "grapefruit juice only," can mess up your body so badly that it just doesn't have any other choice but to lose weight. For healthy weight loss, a moderate dietary approach must be combined with exercise, keeping in mind not to overdo either respect. Two basic concepts will help you to understand this:

Concept 1: When three groups of normal-weight people, with the same habits, weight, and background, are put on a diet that gives them all the same number of calories, one group will gain, one will stay the same, and one will lose weight. This is due to biochemical individuality and differences in metabolism. Be sure and make allowances for your own body needs.

Concept 2: Once a person has determined the daily caloric intake on which he or she neither gains nor loses weight, the effect of food and exercise will be as follows:

Food: An increase causes weight gain, a decrease causes weight loss.

Exercise: An increase causes weight loss, a decrease causes weight gain.

Best results, naturally, are achieved by a combination of both methods.

Exercise and Emotions

"Dieting fads can drive you crazy," says Dr. E. Cheraskin, chairman of the Department of Oral Medicine at the University of Alabama. The fact that insufficient nutrients can affect your mental state is now well established. Dr. Cheraskin explains that emotional disturbances can occur when brain cells aren't getting the substances they need.

At the Mayo Clinic a group of emotionally healthy women was subjected to a popular reducing diet, and soon their emotional stability changed. They experienced anxiety, became hostile, and even felt persecuted. Their overall behavior was very much like that of a group of neurotics.

At the University of Minnesota a group of healthy men was subjected to such a diet, restricting their caloric intake to 1,500 calories per day, and soon they became emotionally unstable, apathetic, irritable, and antisocial.

Is Dieting Enough?

Dr. William Zuti of Kent State University demonstrated the necessity of doing exercise while losing weight in an interesting experiment. Taking a cross-section of single and married women who were overweight and wanted to lose weight, he

61

divided them into three groups and gave each a somewhat different treatment. After 16 weeks, all of them had lost about 11 pounds, but there were some important differences in their physical well being.

In Group 1 the women's caloric intake was reduced by 500 calories per day, and they were not asked to do exercises. After sixteen weeks, it was found that they had lost some fat, but had also lost a lot of lean muscle tissue, the stuff that gives you a good shape. They were lighter but somewhat flabby.

In Group 2 the women were asked to exercise the equivalent of 250 calories per day, and their caloric intake was also reduced by 250 calories. These women lost mainly fat tissue, because the exercise prevented the loss of muscle tissue.

In Group 3 the exercise was increased to burn up 500 calories per day; the women ate normally. As a result, not only did they lose only fat tissue, but they got closer to their peak of physical condition.

THE TOTAL WEIGHT LOSS APPROACH

1. Find your caloric maintenance level: the amount of food you can eat and neither gain nor lose weight. If calculating it in terms of calories is too difficult for you, just let experience be your guide.

2. Follow the rules of good nutrition outlined in Chapter 3. Eat high-quality foods, low in fats, with enough protein, and lots of fresh and unprocessed complex carbohydrates.

3. Don't take drugs to regulate your appetite.

4. Reduce your food intake just a little bit: enough to cause a slight weight loss, but not so much you get uptight about it.

5. Increase your exercise level. Walk the stairs instead of taking the elevator, go for a walk before work, at lunch, and after work. Just be more active wherever you can.

6. Take vitamin and mineral supplements as explained in Chapter 14. This way you can lose weight while getting younger.

7. Go for an extended walk right after every meal; this is especially important for people with hypoglycemia or diabetes.

Weight Gain

So far, nobody has ever established a connection between being underweight and a shorter lifespan.

To gain weight one should follow the same supernutrition rules as outlined earlier. Stuffing yourself with fat foods is absolutely wrong. Superb nutrition in combination with physical therapy gives best results; Rheo Blair, a noted Los Angeles nutrition consultant, has demonstrated this with a high degree of success.

In some cases, if everything else fails, an underweight person can consider the use of organ-specific concentrates as explained in Chapter 15.

Chapter 5

Not for Smokers Only

The children of smokers have been
found to be clumsier, less coordinated,
and slower to learn than the children of
nonsmokers.

	The "Not for Smokers Only" Quiz	Yes	No
1.	Do you smoke cigarettes?	—	—
2.	More than 5 cigarettes per day?	—	—
3.	More than 10 cigarettes per day?	—	—
4.	Do you prefer cigarettes with filters and low levels of tar and nicotine?	—	—
5.	Do you often inhale other people's cigarette smoke?	—	—
6.	If you smoke cigars, or a pipe, do you inhale the smoke?	—	—
7.	Do you have, or is there a history of the following in your family: heart disease, cancer, respiratory problems?	—	—
8.	Do you take additional vitamins E and C for protection against cigarette smoke?	—	—
9.	If a smoker, are you aware of the effects

of cigarette smoke on your health and are
you making every effort to quit?   — —

If you answered "yes" to questions 1 and 3, don't even
think of skipping this chapter.

If you don't smoke and answered "no" to question 5, you
can safely go to the next chapter.

If you don't smoke but answered "yes" to 5 and "no" to 8,
move to the next chapter but try to stay away from the smoke;
it *can* affect your health.

If you answered "yes" to 1, 2, 8, and 9 (with a "no" to 3),
you might skip to the next chapter but come back if you have
difficulties quitting.

Smoking is one subject on which virtually all the experts
agree: It's not good for you. Just how dangerous it is has been
demonstrated over and over in studies involving both laboratory animals and humans. Increased risk of lung cancer is just
one of the possible consequences; others include cardiovascular disorders, decreased endurance, hormonal imbalances,
and a huge drain on the pocketbook. All these items add up
to a major factor in shortening a person's lifespan.

Why Quit Smoking?

Now that the hazards of smoking have been proven conclusively, smokers should face the facts, evaluate the risks, and
decide if they really want to continue to jeopardize their lives.
However, as so many have discovered, it's not so easy to break
a habit.

If you are a nonsmoker, you might remind your smoker
friends of the negative effects of cigarettes, but don't bug
them all the time; this only gets them stubborn and upset. I
face this situation all the time, and it's painful to see how some

of my friends are literally killing themselves. But I also remember what a pain a nagging nonsmoker was to me when I still smoked. So, let's just take a cold look at some facts, and let the smokers decide for themselves.

"Strong evidence now indicates that it isn't only the nicotine and tar in cigarette smoke that can be lethal. So can the gases." This was the opening statement in a magnificent article in *Reader's Digest,* October 1976, that revealed the effects of carbon monoxide and other toxic gases on the incidence of heart disease and other health problems. So please, don't assume you're safe if you smoke cigarettes that are low in tar and nicotine, even though they are a bit better than regular ones.

MORE RESEARCH DATA ON SMOKING CIGARETTES

Among other recent findings related to smoking are the following:

Dr. Oscar Auerbach, cell cytologist, estimated that if you are over 40 and smoke about two packs per day, your chance of getting lung cancer can be 2,000 percent higher than that of a nonsmoker. In fact, cigarette smokers have higher rates of literally every cancer, especially bladder cancer.

Dr. Henry Sullivan writes in the March 1973 issue of *Geriatrics* that the lung cancer survival rate, after all possible treatments, is only about 7 percent.

Intelligence is also affected. In England, Professor James Butler tested the 7-year-old children of smokers and discovered that, with only a few exceptions, they were clumsier than the children of nonsmokers, had an impaired spatial sense, and, with only a few exceptions, were in the lower 10 percent of their class.

Dr. David Burns, a researcher for the U.S. Government's

National Clearing House on Smoking and Health, explains why your vision is also affected and why this can cause higher rates of automobile accident: "The eyes need a lot of oxygen which they get from blood. The nicotine in cigarettes causes the blood vessels in the eyes to contract so that they carry less blood and therefore less oxygen."

That peripheral vision is reduced by long-term cigarette smoking was shown by Dr. Norman Heimstra of the University of South Dakota.

Andrudh K. Jain, a research analyst of the Population Council, reported data which showed that women over 30 who smoke more than 15 cigarettes per day in addition to taking birth control pills, die of heart attacks or blood clots nearly 12 times more frequently than those who do not smoke.

In other studies researchers showed that it was possible to cause lung cancer in animals by exposing them to the tar products of only five cigarettes, that a definite correlation existed between wrinkle formation and the number of cigarettes smoked, and that cigarette smoking can affect hormone levels and lead to impotence in older men. A pregnant woman who smokes also has a higher chance of having a stillborn baby than a pregnant nonsmoker. And if the smoker's child lives, it will weigh less than the child of a nonsmoker.

Why Don't We Hear About These Facts More Often?

A few years ago a friend asked me to write an article on aging for his magazine. I did, and when I showed him the piece he immediately returned it to me with the remark: "Do you think I want to kill myself? If I print this, I probably won't get any cigarette advertising money."

It appears that at least part of the printed media is worried about losing advertising money if they say something against cigarette smoking. They are probably right. Why bite the hand that feeds you?

I, for one, am not against cigarette advertising, but I think we should emphasize honesty in the ads. Naturally you don't get sexier or more attractive if you smoke, but if someone wants to kill himself, isn't this his or her own choice? Let people make their own decisions. Hundreds of years ago it was mainly the stronger one who survived; today it's the more intelligent one.

How to Quit

There are many ways to quit smoking, but all rely on the same basic theory. When we reach for a cigarette, something up in our head tells us that this is what we need—whether because advertising has gotten to us, or we are seeking the approval of our peer group, or emulating an authority figure who smokes, or whatever. No matter what the excuses are, if we really want to quit we have to convince ourselves, directly and indirectly, that there is absolutely nothing good in smoking cigarettes.

It can be done by unbrainwashing yourself. I quit by forcing myself to read an article on the bad effects of cigarette smoking once for every five cigarettes I smoked.

It can be also achieved by letting other professionals do the brainwashing on you. The Schick Centers, Smokers Anonymous, and many other organizations will help in your efforts. Most of these withdrawal methods are based on the principle of giving you a very small annoyance every time you smoke. Often you don't consciously recognize the nuisance, but your brain registers it. After doing this for a while, gradually increasing the annoyance, there will come a time when you reach for a cigarette and your brain will tell you not to smoke. It works!

TIPS TO HELP YOU TO QUIT

1. Smoke only half the cigarette. The remaining half acts as a filter, and you get only about ¼ the tar and nicotine into your lungs. Even if this means you smoke more cigarettes, you will be ahead.

2. Smoke filter cigarettes and cigarettes low in tar and nicotine.

3. When you get the urge to light up, ask yourself if you can't wait another 5 to 10 minutes. This should reduce the number of cigarettes you smoke per day.

4. If you hear or read about some new and devastating research findings about smoking, don't ignore it. Get all the information you can, and force yourself to read any article on this subject at least twice. Let your brain do the judging.

5. When you see a particularly appealing advertisement, just remember that the models are appearing in the ad for money. They might not be smokers themselves and would probably give you the same convincing smile if they were asked to promote any other product. Keep in mind that somebody wants to make a profit on you, and that the money you spend on cigarettes could amount to as much as $300,000 by the time you retire if you invested it in safe bonds starting at the age of 20.

6. If you gained weight during previous efforts to quit, this time try changing to the low-fat and low-sugar diet suggested in chapter 3 when you stop smoking.

If You Must Smoke

There are large numbers of people who have, or have not, evaluated the risks of smoking and plan to continue their habit. Either they feel that their risk is not so high, or they are not strong enough to quit, or they just love it so much that they don't care what happens to their health, sex life, and looks.

In order to reduce the risk to the lowest possible level while you continue to smoke, there are a few things you can do.

Again, smoke only half the cigarette, as explained above. Even if you smoke more cigarettes, the overall amounts of tar and nicotine that reach your lungs will be reduced.

Try to keep the number of cigarettes smoked as low as possible.

Smoke cigarettes that are low in tar and nicotine. A study released by the Department of Health recently showed that this can lower (but not eliminate) your health risks.

Use additional filters for even better results.

Protect yourself with antioxidants.

ANTIOXIDANT PROTECTION

Smoking cigarettes subjects your body to large amounts of materials which oxidize (combine with oxygen) and destroy living tissue. Several of these substances—known as oxides, a type of oxidant—are found in cigarette smoke. They are formed when the tobacco and the cigarette paper is burned, and it is now believed that their effect on our health is as bad as the tar and nicotine in cigarettes.

Vitamins C and E and very small amounts of the trace mineral selenium (found in special types of brewer's yeast, garlic, and some other plants, depending on its presence as nutrient in the soil) are antioxidants and can protect you to some degree. I have demonstrated this value in a longevity study with mice, but the protective effect was not 100 percent. Animals given vitamin supplements fared better than those receiving no extra antioxidant, but not as well as nonsmokers.

Vitamin A has recently received extensive recognition in

cancer treatment and prevention. The mechanism by which all these vitamins act is not yet well understood. They might all work as antioxidants or they might help in stimulating immune responses. One thing is for sure: They help and they are very important.

Vitamin A is found in multivitamin formulations in quantities of 10,000 international units. However, if you are thinking of increasing your dose of vitamin A, be sure to read chapter 14 and the Table of Precautions that follows it. It has been estimated that each cigarette smoked destroys about 20 mg of vitamin C; adjust your vitamin C intake accordingly. Supplementation with vitamin E and the trace mineral selenium is also suggested, but quantities have not yet been established.

Certain sulfur-amino acids, as found in egg protein, are also good antioxidants and have been included in special vitamin formulations for smokers.

Other factors, like air pollution or perhaps chemicals you work with, act in a synergistic way in cancer formation. One risk factor increases the other. Try to reduce your risk by eliminating as many of these contributing factors as possible. For example, asbestos workers can get lung cancer from inhaling asbestos fibers, but their risk increases by 800 percent if combined with cigarette smoking.

THE RIGHT OF OTHERS TO BREATHE CLEAN AIR

And, if you decide to continue smoking, please allow nonsmokers the right to inhale clean air. Think of something that is highly repulsive to you, something that not only annoys you but makes you ill as well. That's the way most nonsmokers feel about cigarette smoking. Please understand.

In talking about marijuana, the only question is "how much?" Large amounts will naturally also subject your body to tar products and carbon monoxide; therefore the health risk is again increased. Large amounts have also been shown to affect people's sleep level. During a normal sleep period one reaches down into the fourth stage, which gives the most restful rest. After smoking grass one doesn't reach this stage of sleep and therefore wakes up in the morning with the feeling, "Am I tired! I could sleep another five hours."

In rare cases marijuana has been shown to affect hormone levels in the blood in men and actually caused the development of breasts. It is now believed that even medium amounts can cause hormonal changes in men and therefore possibly lead to impotence.

Small amounts, however—a few puffs once or twice per week—appear to have little or no effect on a person's health; for some it might be even helpful as an aid to relaxation.

Rather than smoking one or two packs of regular cigarettes, I must say that I would rather see my friends take a few puffs of marijuana. But the best solution of all is to inhale nothing but clean, fresh air!

Chapter 6

The Environmental Factors

Despite the tough 1972 amendment to the Federal Water Pollution Control Act, a recent study of water supplies in 80 cities showed that most contained contaminated water.

Time, October 20, 1975

In an age in which we have the technology to build experimental automobile engines that give 270 miles per gallon, to work out practical aspects of recycling waste materials, to build clean energy self-sufficient homes, and to develop greenhouses in which plants seeded in the morning can yield a crop at night, it is ironic that the "environmental disease" —pollution at every level—is becoming the health problem of the century.

Numerous scientific studies have shown that clean air and water not only promote longevity but are essential requirements for health. Industrialized, highly polluted areas in this country have higher rates of diseases such as cancer, atherosclerosis, arteriosclerosis, and emphysema. People living there also have an accelerated rate of aging, and their average life-spans are decreased.

Congress is faced frequently with decisions on measures to help clean the environment. Unfortunately, there is a great deal of opposition by the dirty-air lobby, and the big clean up is still far away. We have the technology to do the job, but political pressure holds us back. Politicians talk about pollution, officials in our government express concern, bills are introduced; but in the end, the big polluters always seem to wind up with the advantage. The equilibrium between health and pollution has not yet shifted toward health.

On Our Air

Inhaling asbestos particles has long been known to contribute to lung cancer, and when combined with cigarette smoking it can increase the lung cancer risk by 800 percent. Our current precautions against getting this material into the air are insufficient. Even when it is used on a small scale in repairing things in the home, masks and filters should be used. The cells in our lungs that normally digest and dispose of inhaled particles act very strangely when they encounter asbestos; they tumble back and forth as if they were drunk. They have no means of effectively disposing of the asbestos fibers.

Oxidants in the air pollution start adverse reactions in our bodies that lead to the formation of molecules which the chemist calls "free radicals." These free radicals can cause great damage to living tissue, and in specific reactions they have been proposed as factors in cancer formation (for details read *Supernutrition for Healthy Hearts* by Richard Passwater). The pollutants we are concerned about are carbon monoxide, the nitrogen and sulfur oxides, and ozone. Besides these gases, we have solid particles in air pollution.

VINYL CHLORIDE

This raw material used in the manufacture of PVC-plastic, is another possible factor in cancer formation. Ironically, this plastic is frequently used in food containers and wrappings. It is my opinion that PVC should not be used for these purposes until we have established that it is safe. But cancer isn't the only danger in vinyl chloride; birth defects is another. In several areas of the United States where polyvinyl chloride is manufactured, it was found that women bore a remarkably higher number of children with abnormalities. These findings were confirmed by researchers in Russia and Germany. Producers of PVC sometimes argue that cleaning the environment in which these people live would put them out of work; not a very convincing line of reasoning to me. What is more important, economics or health?

HEAVY METALS

Children living near industrial smelters have higher lead levels in their blood, and this is especially dangerous because children have less resistance to the toxic effects of lead poisoning than do adults. Overall higher lead levels in all ages have also been observed in people who live close to expressways with heavy traffic. Lead inhibits certain enzyme systems in our body and can cause other disorders.

AIR POLLUTION FROM AUTOMOBILES

Most air pollution is caused by automobiles. However, according to a report by the Champion Spark Plug Company, more than half of this type of pollution is created by automobiles that are not properly maintained or well tuned. Testing was done at shopping centers and parking lots where emission levels of cars were checked by a team of mechanics. Of the cars tested, 21 percent produced 55 percent of the carbon monoxide pollution, and 27 percent of the cars produced 58 percent of the hydrocarbon emissions.

"This situation is largely due to cars being undermaintained by their owners. We feel emissions inspection on a regular basis is the most effective way to reduce automotive air pollution," said David L. Walker, the company's director of automotive technical services.

A third type of pollution caused by automobiles is nitrogen oxide emissions. Oxidation reactions that destroy living tissue are the major problems with this type of pollution.

OFFSHORE OIL DRILLING AND OIL TERMINALS

The air pollution in the Los Angeles area will soon be increased by offshore drilling. According to Air Resources Board chief Tom Quinn in California, the offshore oil drilling will add pollution in the equivalent of 900,000 automobiles to the already highly contaminated air.

The Air Resources Board of California reported that a proposed Long Beach supertanker terminal for receiving Alaskan oil would add the pollution equivalent of 2.7 million cars to the air in this area.

Californians living close to the beach and paying highly for the privilege of inhaling relatively clean air will now get their air "preconditioned." Not only will the air be more polluted, but the weather along the shoreline will also be strongly affected. More particles in the air means more fog and clouds. Will the sun along the California beaches become a memory of the past?

The same problems exist in other areas of the United States, particularly the East Coast and the Gulf of Mexico, where offshore oil drilling and other oil-related projects are planned. Regulations for this type of business are very vague, and restrictions are few. Clean air is not yet a reality; it's a futuristic dream. And many polluters are working hard to keep it this way.

What Can Be Done Immediately?

In most cities, including Los Angeles, I would estimate, based on published figures, that air pollution could be reduced by at least 50 percent within six months if we would all take part of the responsibility and initiate the following steps:

1. Use the media (radio, TV, newspapers, magazines) to educate people as to the dangers of pollution, and the importance of doing something about it. We must make people conscious that clean air requires a concerted approach, and that each person's contribution counts.

2. Make automobile tune-ups mandatory at predetermined time intervals. Highway pollution control checks should enforce the law. Increase the fines for disconnecting pollution devices and for driving undermaintained cars. Let everybody know that the minor savings through the violation of these laws will definitely be offset by fines if they are caught. I estimate that this measure alone could reduce air pollution by 20 to 40 percent, depending on the degree of enforcement.

3. Add methanol to the fuel of our automobiles in amounts from 15 to 30 percent. Methanol is a clean-burning alcohol that is available from several industrial branches. It can be added to the gas without harmful effects to the engine. We are already using it as "dry gas" as an additive to gasoline in states where it gets very cold during the winter; it picks up

moisture and thus avoids freezing of gas lines. The gasoline lobby's claim that this modification would result in excessive cost increases to the consumer is a political argument not supported by unbiased research. But we do have evidence that an air pollution reduction of up to 20 percent could come about from this measure.

4. Put NOX (pollution control) devices on the engines of older cars. True, these pollution control devices reduce mileage to a small degree, but people who don't like this could be offered the option of installing a special type of ignition system that reduces pollution but increases mileage. This new ignition system costs a little more but if its purchase were tax deductible, the burden would be small. Another 10 percent reduction in pollution would be a certainty.

5. Enforce our current antipollution laws. For example, we could establish a helicopter patrol to sample air above industrial plants and assure that air-pollution devices are not only installed but switched on and working. Fines for pollution violators have been very low and are often cancelled when companies agreed to install clean-air devices. A tougher attitude with more and bigger fines would make quite a difference. Since all this depends on the type of industries and on the number of plants in one specific area, one can only estimate the reduction in pollution; guesses vary from 10 to 30 percent.

6. Put a tax on automobiles with big engines but make sure that the money generated by these and other measures is used to improve air quality.

7. Educate people about some basic health concepts. It takes a lot of gasoline to take the car to the local drugstore or supermarket. On the other hand, a short walk would be very beneficial. We should encourage the use of car pools, but we can't force people to participate. We all pay highway taxes and should have equal rights to use our roads.

8. Almost every utility pole that carries high voltage electricity produces some ozone; you can see and hear it if you take a walk any evening when the humidity is high. Sparks up to several inches long between oppositely-charged wires or between the wires and metal towers supporting them can cause ozone to form; that's how we make this gas in the laboratory. Better insulation on electric poles and slightly lower voltage would help reduce the amount of ozone in the air. At very high altitudes, ozone acts as a shield against ultraviolet radiation and is an important component of our atmosphere. But in our immediate environment, ozone is a highly toxic gas that can do serious damage to living tissues. Increasing the ozone levels in our cities will have no effect on atmospheric ozone and can only be harmful to us.

9. Educate people about the use of solar energy. Give tax credits for installing such devices. Make public funds available to assist in installing them in highly polluted areas. Local and state governments should set examples by installing solar devices in every new building, and in each old one when it is remodeled. A trend toward efficiency would help reduce the taxpayer's load and improve the environment.

10. Intercorporate transportation, where trucks owned by one company could carry loads for others, was suggested by the General Accounting Office in Washington. This practice would save fuel and reduce pollution caused by diesel engines. It was found that empty trucks often traveled thousands of miles returning from runs.

Following these simple steps would mean that we could see the mountains every day in the Los Angeles area, that you wouldn't smell Chicago from 20 miles away, and that flying over New York would give us a view of more than a few tall buildings sticking their tops out of the haze.

For your personal program, if you live in polluted air, there is really only one solution: Move out. Air quality is improving but very, very slowly. Installing air purifiers in your house or office will help somewhat.

For your long-term survival, keep a close eye on what is happening to the environment around you. Let your government representatives know how you feel about things, and keep a record of how they vote on environmental issues. You might consider joining a concerned citizens' group that follows the voting records of politicians. And if you find a bad apple don't just vote against him, work actively against him.

The Water We Drink

In the seventeenth and eighteenth centuries, American cities were hit hard by typhoid fever, yellow fever, diphtheria, and other diseases. In 1699, about 6 percent of the population of Philadelphia was wiped out; in 1793, another epidemic killed about 10 percent of the inhabitants. Five years later, when the same thing happened again, about 80 percent of the population fled.

Medical advisers could not agree on what caused these epidemics. Some blamed a tropical disease brought into the country on ships; others attributed the problem to unsanitary conditions and unsafe water supplies. The city authorities, wanting to make sure, followed several types of advice and eventually the fever disappeared.

Perhaps the most effective of all the measures the city took was the construction of a public water system. Steam engines were installed to pump water from the river, then the best source for clean water, into the city through large wooden pipes.

The Philadelphia system was a big step forward in supplying city dwellers with clean water; other cities soon followed this example.

WHERE DO WE STAND TODAY?

Some people claim that our water is absolutely safe; others fear that it can cause cancer and other diseases. Before examining this important controversy, let's take a look at why a good water supply is so important for our health.

More than 60 percent of our body consists of water. All metabolic reactions going on inside us are based on this life-supporting liquid, and without it life as we know it would be impossible. Our body fluids, which are mainly water, carry nutrients to our cells and get rid of waste materials by carrying them to the kidney, which filters out what our body wants to get rid of.

Any toxic material that gets into our body fluids is immediately distributed throughout our body and thus can affect every organ system. Since a large percentage of our food consists of water, and since we also drink quite a bit of water, anything in it will also wind up in our body fluids. The only safety valves our body can use to get rid of toxic materials are the liver and our immune system. But they are effective only to a certain degree and, as explained later, it is extremely important not to overload them.

WHAT EVERYONE SHOULD KNOW
ABOUT CITY WATER

More than 18 years ago the Reserve Mining Company began processing taconite northeast of Duluth, on Lake Superior. Daily 67,000 tons of wastes were dumped into the lake. A significant portion of the waste consisted of cummingtonite, an asbestos-like material.

Because asbestos is a proven cause of cancer, Dr. Irving

Selikoff, a specialist on environmental cancer factors, suggested that people shouldn't drink Lake Superior water. Dr. Cuyler Hammond of the American Cancer Society said he would not drink from Duluth's reservoir. Dr. Phillip Cook of the EPA, writing in *Today's Health,* said: "I won't even let my wife shampoo the rug with it. We know this material can go from the water into the air, and we know you can't get it out once it's in you."

Examinations of Duluth's drinking water showed that it contained from 10 to 100 times greater amounts of asbestos-like fibers than normal public water supplies.

Only in 1976 and '77 were agreements worked out with the EPA to stop this pollution, and dumping grounds were assigned to the mining company. This is an example of the lack of true concern for the environment by certain industries. The dangers of what they were, and in many cases are still, doing were known many years ago. Only after strong actions by governmental agencies were results achieved. Shouldn't every branch of industry honestly examine itself and do everything possible to eliminate pollution, instead of just seeing what it can get away with?

But Duluth isn't the only city with these lethal materials in its drinking water. Preliminary findings indicate that people in New York, Philadelphia, Atlanta, Chicago, Boston, Dallas, Kansas City, Denver, San Francisco, and Seattle are exposed to them as well.

THE MAJOR PROBLEMS WITH OUR WATER

The U.S. Senate Select Committee on National Water Resources divided water pollutants into eight major groups. Let us take a look at them and their effects:

1. *Sewage and other oxygen-demanding wastes:* These are largely organic compounds that can be biodegraded by microorganisms, but the breakdown process requires oxygen. If too much sewage is dumped into a river or lake, this uses all the oxygen, leaving none for fish and plant life, which then die. Since many communities draw water from these sources, the high bacterial growth—and the extra chlorine many cities use to kill that growth—can cause health problems.

2. *Infectious agents:* Bacteria and viruses from human and animal waste are the main sources but there are many others, including slaughtering houses and decaying animals.

3. *Plant nutrients:* Nitrogen and phosphorus compounds can increase undesired algal growth, which can result in lower oxygen levels in the water, again leading to the death of a body of water. Nitrates are very dangerous because they can oxidize other nitrogen compounds into nitrose-compounds (cancer-causing chemicals).

4. *Exotic organic chemicals:* These include pesticides, detergents, aromatic compounds, oil products, and others. Exotic organic chemicals are both extremely dangerous and relatively difficult to remove from the water. Some of them can be carcinogens. To illustrate this point, Drs. Wilhelm Hueper and William Payne from the National Cancer Institute extracted some of the water from a polluted river, removed the organic chemicals, and tested them on mice. Cancers developed in several of the animals but not in the control group.

The next question they had to answer was: Were these chemicals still present in the water after it passed through a local water treatment plant? Sure enough, even the treated water contained chemicals that could cause tumors.

5. *Inorganic minerals and chemical compounds:* Besides minerals important for life processes, like calcium and magnesium, we also find highly hazardous minerals like mercury and lead in our drinking water. The amount of lead has increased

dramatically due to leaded gasolines. Anything that goes into the air will ultimately find its way into our waterways. These minerals can be removed by the right methods, but often the procedures used are not good enough.

6. *Sediments:* Soil and mineral particles reduce the amount of sunlight that penetrates the water and cover spawning grounds and food supplies for aquatic life. When oxidized, these particles also remove oxygen from the water, reducing the amount available for animal life.

7. *Radioactive compounds:* These arise mainly from nuclear reactors, but also from nuclear tests and from other radioactive materials used by research scientists. The precautions taken in this field could stand some improvements. The radioactive waste from nuclear reactors is increasing by thousands of tons every year and is becoming a real problem. Storage areas are never 100 percent safe. Suggestions that this material may enter the environment through some kind of accident are not so far-fetched.

Nuclear energy once looked very promising; today its dangers far outweigh its advantages. Any newly allocated research money should go for the ultimate: clean and pollution-free solar-energy programs.

8. *Heat:* Power plants withdraw water from rivers and lakes for cooling purposes and return it a few degrees warmer. The higher water temperature increases algal growth and thus removes oxygen at a higher rate. In addition, oxygen is less soluble in water at higher temperatures, and so depletion of oxygen is accelerated.

BETTER HEALTH THROUGH CLEANER WATER

Purifying our water supplies should be an absolute top priority. It isn't that we don't know how to do it; we are just lazy and careless. Like people who smoke cigarettes, we are all risking our health continuously, but since we don't get cancer or show other ill effects when we drink tap water, we assume it doesn't hurt us in the long run.

The steps our water facility engineers can take include better quality control, final fine-filtering, less chlorination, and passing drinking water through beds of activated charcoal. Charcoal is inexpensive, it removes the exotic organic chemicals, and it protects us from toxic chemicals just in case a spill should introduce a larger quantity into our water supplies. Algae formation on activated carbon used to be a problem, but several methods have been developed to deal with it.

Removal of heavy metals like lead and mercury from the water is often very difficult, and the degree of removal is unsatisfactory. Making sure that these metals don't get into the water supply in the first place is our best protection. What else can we do about that? Not much, but there is one experiment which might point us in the right direction. Drs. M. Mokranjac and C. Petrovic, when they were at the University of Paris, France, in 1964, studied the effect of mercury poisoning on guinea pigs to determine possible ways of preventing the poisoning. They found that animals that received large doses of vitamin C survived mercury poisoning at levels that were fatal to animals without the extra vitamin C intake. The amounts of vitamin C given were equivalent to about 14 grams in a human.

Fluoridation of drinking water is another issue that is often misunderstood. Because fluorine is an essential element, some health officials favor fluoridation of our water supplies. They appear to overlook the fact that the level of fluoride intake is critical, and that larger amounts will interfere seriously with enzyme systems in our body. Our intake of fluoride is already above our needs, and this is probably one of the reasons why there is already a well established link between

fluoridation and cancer. Before we dump any more questionable materials into our water, we should try to clean up the
impurities in it.

WHAT CAN YOU DO ABOUT YOUR DRINKING WATER?

1. For starters, limit your intake of tap water and substitute
good drinking water or a high-quality mineral water whenever
possible. Several companies are making water filters that can
be attached to the water faucet. Activated carbon removes
organic chemicals and chlorine (also suspected of causing
cancer), and a microfilter removes solid impurities. Different
models of the Instapure water filter by Water Pik can be
attached to the faucet and cost from $20 to $30. A larger, very
sophisticated water purifier, with a 6-stage hermetically
sealed system for which no refills have to be bought, is made
by Cal-Hurley (P.O. Box 484, Canoga Park, California 91305)
and sells for about $130.

2. Encourage your local authorities to review the water
purification projects in your area. Suggest that they not use
fluoridation and do use carbon and microfiltration.

3. Let your government representatives know that you want
them to enact legislature for a clean environment. Complain
to local pollution control agencies about violations you observe. If you make a complaint, your local authorities must
follow up and should report back to you. The same goes for
air pollution violations.

4. Don't drink distilled water unless you have thoroughly
evaluated its quality. Often it is made from regular tap water
and, due to a process called steam distillation, the exotic
organic chemicals can be carried over into the distillate. The
problem could be solved by distilling water which first has

been purified with a carbon filter. I personally do not recommend distilled water because valuable minerals like calcium and magnesium have been removed from it; in studies on humans these minerals have been found to be very important for the prevention of heart disease.

Water softeners also remove calcium and magnesium and they often add sodium to the water instead. Because sodium is a possible cause of high blood pressure, the use of "softened" drinking water cannot be recommended.

Chapter 7

Alcohol and Other Drugs

Since alcohol is, in a sense, both a food
and a drug, it can in both roles affect
our weight, our sex life, and our appearance.

Morris Chafetz, M.D.
in *Why Drinking Can Be
Good For You*

The Drinking Person's Quiz

If you drink at all, a simple test that is completely private
can indicate whether you have an alcohol problem: Can you
abstain from all drinking—wine, beer, and hard liquor—for
six days in a row?

Don't just ask yourself the question, answer it by actually
going for six days without a drink. If you worry about what
your friends might think if you don't drink with them, order
something that looks like an alcoholic drink, or just tell them
you're on a diet that doesn't allow you to drink. If you are a
health-oriented person, you may not have a problem, but
what of your friends and family?

Some Alcohol Statistics

Nearly 10 percent of people who drink are alcoholics or have a serious drinking problem. Alcohol consumption in the United States has reached a new high of 2.6 gallons per year per person. Since approximately 50 percent of our population doesn't drink or drinks very little, the average consumption among drinkers is 5.2 gallons of straight alcohol: The equivalent of approximately 50 quarts of strong liquor, per year.

Half of all killings in the United States are associated with drinking alcohol (either the killer or the victim, and both in many instances, were drinking before the time of death). Half of the automobile deaths (approximately 26,000 per year) involve people that were drinking. If you are a heavy drinker, your chance of being divorced is about 750 percent higher than for a nondrinker or a moderate drinker, and your lifespan is shortened an average of 10 to 12 years.

Alcoholic men used to outnumber alcoholic women by six to one. In some areas of this country, women have caught up with men and the numbers are equal. In every branch of the American economy, management is very concerned about alcohol. According to Richard Gerstenberg, Chairman of General Motors, alcoholics cost U.S. industry about $10 billion per year. Alcoholism committees are being set up in plants all over the country, and recovery programs have produced encouraging results. In a study of 101 Oldsmobile workers, the improvements due to such a program were as follows: There was a 50 percent decrease in lost manhours, 30 percent decline in sickness and accident claims, 63 percent reduction in disciplinary action, and an 82 percent reduction in accidents.

What Does Alcohol Do To Your Body?

"Cheers!" You lift the glass and just a few minutes after your drink goes "down the hatch," its alcohol begins to hit your blood stream. Since alcohol is very high in calories (half a pint of strong liquor like scotch contains about 600 calories), a drink satisfies the body's need for calories, and therefore the heavy drinker has a tremendously reduced appetite. His food intake is decreased, and his intake of essential nutrients falls far below the minimum. Brain cells, which can't store nutrients, depend on a constant supply of them from food. Malnutrition leads to brain damage and deterioration to such a degree that the brains of alcoholics are completely worthless for students of medical research. The more a person drinks, the more he or she replaces essential nutrients with empty calories. The higher the alcohol intake, the higher the degree of possible malnutrition. If, on the other hand, the food intake is enough to supply all the essential nutrients, the excess calories in the alcohol will make you overweight.

There is evidence that good nutrition, including adequate supplies of vitamins, can delay the effects of alcohol and possibly prevent a person from becoming an alcoholic. A nutrition program for people near the borderline of alcoholism can have dramatic results.

Alcohol's damaging effects on the heart are probably due to nutritional deficiencies of the drinker. Heart cells, too, must be constantly bathed in fluids containing a good supply of all nutrients or they are damaged.

The liver is another organ strongly affected by alcohol. At first researchers assumed that only large amounts of alcohol would affect it. However, it has recently been found that three or four drinks per day over a few weeks' period can make the liver fatty and much less efficient. Drs. D. VanThiel, H. Gavaler, and R. Lester have found that vitamin A metabolism, which takes place mainly in the liver, is inhibited by alcohol and this is a possible explanation for the sterility of heavy drinkers among men.

That the typical American diet can make people tend toward alcoholism was demonstrated by Dr. E. Cheraskin, Professor of Medicine at the University of Alabama. In an experiment, rats were fed the equivalents of coffee and doughnuts for breakfast and ham sandwich and Coke for lunch. For dinner, given the choice between water and alcohol as their drinking fluid, these animals preferred alcohol. However, when the same rats received a diet consisting of all required nutrients, vitamins, and minerals, they preferred water.

In other studies, it was found that animals on nutritionally deficient diets consumed several times as much alcohol as animals on good diets. These experiments show that improving the quality of nutrition for alcoholics is essential. Considering that snack foods like soft drinks, potato chips, etc., make up about 28 percent of the American diet, there is good reason for a high rate of alcoholism in the United States.

AMOUNTS OF MISSING NUTRIENTS

To demonstrate how a person's nutrition is upset by adding empty calories, let's use our computer again and calculate some numbers. There are established ranges of essential nutrients, vitamins, and minerals for every person. Macronutrients can be calculated on the basis of the daily caloric expenditure, and vitamins and minerals can be compared to the Recommended Daily Allowance (RDA).

We'll assume that a man or a woman with a daily caloric expenditure of about 2,500 calories is eating a very good diet which supplies the required amounts of macronutrients (protein, complex carbohydrates, fibers, etc.) and 100 percent of the RDA vitamins and minerals.

If this person now starts drinking three mixed drinks per day, the equivalent of about 650 calories, the food intake must be reduced by 650 calories to keep the weight constant. If this person ate as before, without burning up the calories through extra exercises, a weight gain of about 1.3 pounds would occur per week.

Reducing foods in the equivalent of 650 calories per day would now induce a deficiency of all essential nutrients of about 25 percent per day. Since many people drink, and eat junk foods at the same time, it is very well possible that alcohol can greatly contribute to inducing nutritional deficiencies.

The Treatment of Alcoholism

The treatments of this disease are numerous. With many scientists working in this field and treating alcoholics, however, Alcoholics Anonymous (AA) does the best and least expensive job. AA does not use psychiatrists or other professionals; it is just people helping people. Alcoholics and former alcoholics meet to share their experiences and discuss their common goal: to help people recognize that they cannot cope with this problem alone. An AA book called *Alcoholics Anonymous* describes the philosophy of the organization and cites case histories of people who have gone through the program successfully.

Alcoholism treatments available in hospitals include educational films, discussions, aversion therapy, behavior conditioning, and drugs. The cost is usually between $1,000 and $2,000.

One very promising drug, "antabuse," was developed in

Denmark. After taking this compound, one cannot drink alcohol without feeling faint and vomiting. No alcohol consumption, no ill effects. Once experienced, the drug doesn't reduce your desire for alcohol directly, but it certainly prevents you from drinking.

Whether the problem is simple overuse or true alcoholism, one step is necessary before any treatment can be effective: The person must admit to himself (or herself) that the problem exists. Attitude discussions, group counseling, and encounters with other people who have the same problem are very helpful, but they are merely a start. The will to change must grow out of a recognition of the seriousness of the situation.

Since the abused body of a heavy drinker has usually been depleted of many important nutrients, superb nutrition and avoidance of all junk foods and high-fat foods are essential. Then, a prevention-oriented doctor should design a strong supplementation program, based on a precise evaluation of the person's nutrition and other habits. This supplementation must consist of vitamins and minerals, but might also include digestive enzymes and specialty foods. Since the liver has probably been damaged, supplementation with liver concentrates (discussed in Chapter 15) will help.

The Money You Drink To

We often associate drinking with having fun and being happy. For the moderate drinker this is probably true, but one sometimes wonders whether the heavy drinkers are trying to forget how much money they are spending on this health hazard.

A heavy drinker or alcoholic spends about $4,500 per year on alcohol if he does his drinking in bars or restaurants. The long-term drinker will thus have spent, during his entire working lifetime, so much money that he could have accumulated $1.8 million had he invested drinking money in government bonds paying 8.5 percent interest. If he started drinking at the age of 30, he could have accumulated $900,-000 by the time he retires. The average drinker, the one who consumes "only" 50 bottles per year, could have saved $500,-000, assuming that ⅔ of his drinking was done in bars and he started drinking at the age of 22.

So, the next time you lift your glass, think about what is more important: you, your health, money, and life, or the liquor industry's profits?

Rules for Good Drinking

One drink in the company of good friends can be fun and has very little chance of hurting you. Some studies on humans suggest that a reasonable amount of alcohol will actually help lengthen your lifespan. The important factors are where, when, and how you drink. These, and other interesting facts about drinking, are covered by Dr. Morris Chafetz in *Why Drinking Can Be Good For You* (Stein and Day). Here are a few guidelines:

1. Drink alcoholic beverages only when you really have the desire for them; otherwise drink healthy, nonalcoholic drinks.

2. Always try to eat some good food before you drink; this slows the rate at which alcohol enters the blood stream.

3. Dilute your drinks with fruit juice or any other nonalcoholic fluid you like. (Don't use carbonated beverages for this; they make alcohol enter the blood stream faster.)

4. Make yourself comfortable wherever you drink. If you are uncomfortable, and slightly under distress, you are more likely to drink more.

Other "Dangerous Drugs"

Few would deny that alcohol is really just a drug, and a dangerous one which, when abused, belongs somewhere on the same list as barbiturates, amphetamines, and heroin. Incredible as it may sound, though, legitimate prescriptions may cause more ill effects than the substances we commonly call "dangerous drugs." This topic alone could fill a book, but in the rest of this chapter, we will look briefly at the overuse, misuse, and side effects of prescription drugs.

A WORD ABOUT DRUGS

Drugs are fantastic tools to cure diseases and alleviate pain. Many early drugs were isolated from plants, then analyzed by the chemist and synthesized in the laboratory. Quite a few modern drugs are completely new compounds doing their job in eliminating a certain disease even more efficiently than the natural compounds. But our tremendous success in curing diseases with drugs has made us somewhat careless. We overlook the negative side effects which can be quite detrimental in terms of long-term health.

Almost every drug has side effects. These range all the way from slight discomfort to death. Yet we still use these drugs. Why? Assume a person has caught a disease. If there are no other ways to cure the disease, we must use a drug.

If we know a lot about the disease, how it works, and how we can interfere with it, then we will probably be able to cure it with a small amount of a drug which has very minor side effects. Sounds good? Yes, but that's not the way it really works. Drugs are often prescribed because a pharmaceutical distributor has a tremendous effect on the entire drug market.

Good drug salesmen push hard with whatever they have to sell, the industry spends vast amounts of money reaching doctors with its advertising, and there have even been reports of kickbacks in the marketing of drugs. Doctors often try to justify large prescriptions by saying they want to make sure the disease is cured. In other cases doctors prescribe drugs that are not necessary at all, or prescribe a very expensive drug when a much less expensive one would do the job. Investigators have estimated that this "over-prescription" costs American consumers about $200 million per year.

OVERUSE OF DRUGS

Any drug should be considered dangerous unless proven otherwise. In any case, we should use drugs only when absolutely necessary. To expect the medical profession to deliver perfect health for a certain fee is one of the biggest mistakes we can make. Medicine can help us overcome a disease, but it certainly does not deliver health in the form of a prescription. Since the human species is extremely lazy, people will often choose to "buy health in a bottle" instead of exercising and making other efforts to stay healthy. But good health is not so easily come by and, in many cases, all the drugs in the world could do little for someone who has permitted his body to decay.

Overuse of drugs is widespread, even in our best hospitals. A Senate Health Subcommittee recently heard evidence that at least 50 percent of American prescriptions, especially for antibiotics, were either unnecessary or otherwise incorrect.

This over-prescription was documented by Charles C. Edwards, Assistant Secretary of Health at HEW, and by James V. Visconti of the Ohio State University College of Pharmacy. Edwards and Visconti surveyed 1,045 patients, of whom 340 had received antibiotics. A physician and pharmacist review team judged 13 percent of the prescriptions "rational," 65 percent "irrational," and 22 percent "questionable."

Edward S. Brady, Associate Dean of the University of Southern California School of Pharmacy, said: "It is wasteful to spend money on something that is really not needed, and even a conservative estimate would place . . . over-use and over-purchase of drugs at about 50 percent of the elderly consumer's total drug and health product budget." And, he said, many health professionals treating elderly patients assume that when a drug is prescribed, it is automatically prescribed for the remainder of the patient's life.

Even after a disorder is cured, many patients try to have their prescriptions refilled because they believe they are doing something good for their health by continuing to take the drug. In fact, drug-induced side effects often lead to the exact opposite of good health.

Nonprescription drugs like aspirin, antihistamines, antacids, laxatives, and many others also have side effects. Their overuse can induce serious health problems and hide signs of disorders that need medical attention.

For many, drug overuse begins in childhood, with unnecessary prescriptions for "hyperactivity." One of the most common forms of drug overuse today is the thoughtless prescription of "ritalin" and other substances that will mask hyperactivity in children while threatening to cause dozens of side effects far more serious than the original condition. Just as bad, the reckless dispensing of hyperactivity drugs teaches children to "pop a pill" whenever they suffer from one or another bothersome symptom. That we have safer, more effective alternatives to the drug-based approach has been demonstrated many times, perhaps most clearly by Sidney Walker, M. D., in his article in the December 1974 issue of *Psychology Today*.

Drug-Induced Problems

The more drugs you take, the more frequently you will have adverse reactions; to show this we don't even have to do long-term studies. L.E. Cluff of the University of Florida School of Medicine, Gainsville, recently studied adverse drug reactions of patients in a hospital and found that among 900 patients, 115 harmful reactions occurred. Ninety-seven of the patients experienced their adverse drug reactions while still in the hospital.

Time spent in the hospital due to adverse drug reactions has increased in the past few years. Add to this the fact that every year up to 150,000 people die because of over-prescription, and you have an accurate picture of the ugly side of modern health care.

During a 1976 AMA workshop on human sexuality, held in Tulsa, Dr. Oliver Bjorksten of the South Carolina Medical School at Charleston warned physicians that many drugs can affect human sexual functioning, sometimes leading to impotence in men. The drugs Bjorksten implicated were valium, librium, antihistamines, barbiturates, and medications for asthma, peptic ulcers, digestive disorders, and high blood pressure. Many other drugs are suspected of having similar effects.

THE PILL AND ITS SIDE EFFECTS

A higher rate of cancer and heart disease is associated with taking oral contraceptives. Other disorders that the pill can cause are listed on the information sheet provided by the drug company with each packet, or available from your pharmacist.

Female hormones like diethylstilbesterol (DES), commonly

used in cattle feed to make animals gain weight faster, are part of the "morning after" pill and were given to pregnant women many years ago for other reasons. The powerful long-term effects of drugs was shown by these women's daughters, who are now developing ovarian cancer at a rate much higher than normal. We should investigate this drug much further before we allow it to be sold as a "morning after" pill.

Your New Approach Toward Drugs

1. Make sure you have a prevention-oriented doctor, not one who pulls out his prescription pad whenever you complain about something.

2. Ask your doctor if drugs are truly necessary or if he knows of any nondrug approach which might correct your problem. Follow any nondrug procedure and do everything possible to avoid taking unnecessary drugs.

3. Avoid using nonprescription drugs as much as you can.

4. Don't try to get refills for a prescription unless your doctor specifically tells you to do so.

5. Have your doctor evaluate all the drugs you are taking on a long-term basis.

6. Don't take drugs in front of your children. Don't let them think that pill popping is a normal way of life.

Another drugless approach now practiced by an increasing number of doctors is kinesiology. Testing the strength of specific muscle groups in our bodies gives the doctor clues about internal disorders. Adjustments of the muscles, in combination with organ-specific concentrates, can then make use of drugs unnecessary.

Mark Bricklin's book, *The Practical Encyclopedia of Natural Healing,* outlines many alternatives to surgery and drugs. All the new methods of treatment, including acupuncture, chiropractic techniques, exercise therapy, herbal medicine, osteopathy, and hypnosis are covered in a readable way. If you have any problem that doesn't respond to orthodox treatment, this book will probably have a suggestion for you.

Chapter 8

Stress and How to Handle It

> "Fight always for your highest attainable aim, but never put up resistance in vain."
>
> Dr. Hans Selye
> *The Stress of Life*

The Stress Quiz	Yes	No
1. Are you often under stress?	—	—
2. Does this stress often really get to you?	—	—
3. Is this stress situation mainly at work?	—	—
4. Mainly in your private life?	—	—
5. Do you often grind your teeth and feel you would like to hit somebody?	—	—
6. Do you have high blood pressure?	—	—
7. Do you have a tendency to get ulcers?	—	—
8. Do you drink a lot of coffee?	—	—
9. Do you have a heart problem?	—	—

As you might have guessed, all the correct answers were "no."

If you answered more than two questions "yes": relax! The next time stress gets to you, ask yourself if the accelerated rate of aging is worth all this trouble.

If you answered "yes" to 2 *and* to 6, 7, and/or 9, you have a serious problem with stress. Read this chapter carefully.

We have all heard of examples of the middle-aged business-man who, after becoming extremely excited or upset about something, suffers a heart attack. That psychological stress can bring on heart attacks is generally accepted in medical circles and by the public as well. When a heart does not receive the proper nutrients, and when it is burdened with deposits that contribute to hardening of the arteries, stress becomes especially dangerous.

The true contributing role of stress in heart attacks was discovered by Drs. B. Lown and R. Verrier at the Harvard School of Public Health. These researchers found that when animals were exposed to stressful situations, their hearts showed a relatively high degree of electrical inability, or "fibrillation." In humans, fibrillation is associated with acute heart attacks.

Before we continue, we must redefine stress. We are often under stress, but the effects on different people can vary widely. A general was interviewed and was asked the question: "With your stressful job, don't you get any ulcers?" The general replied: "Me, get ulcers? I give ulcers." Stress, as long as we are capable of handling it, is a very good driving force in our life. However, when stress really gets to you—when you grind your teeth, and when you start telling yourself things that upset you—it changes into distress, and that's what we are trying to avoid. So, stress is O.K., but we want to learn how to handle distress, because that's the bad guy.

What Distress Can Do To You

Distress is also a factor in asthma, arthritis, ulcers, and other diseases. In most cases distress is not the actual cause of physical illness; rather, it picks on the "little guy," making the weakest part of you even weaker. We all have organs or parts of our bodies that are more vulnerable than others, and distress attacks where resistance is lowest.

In the stomach the excretion of gastric juices increases under distress. The higher acidity causes indigestion; stomach muscles knot; tension hampers the movement of foods out of the stomach resulting in more irritation. Repeated distress situations will ultimately lead to an ulcer.

In many people, this type of distress leads to overeating. Perhaps this happens to you. You sit home, unable to concentrate on what you should be doing. Tense and nervous, you cast about for something soothing, fast. Food fits the bill perfectly and is easily available. This nervous eating, of course, leads to overweight, a condition for which higher mortality rates are well established.

Distress also inhibits a healthy and happy sex life. The connection between distress and problems such as frigidity and impotence is known to every psychiatrist. Often sex-related distress starts with a seeming failure or fear of failure, which leads to worry about the next time. Relaxation, so important for enjoyable sex, is incompatible with worry. Result: repeated failure. Thus the situation repeats itself, becoming even more serious.

It is difficult to convince a distressed person that no physical problem is interfering with his or her sexual fulfillment. Lack of knowledge about sex, about the human body, and about proper ways to handle distress contribute to the problem, making sex not only unenjoyable but frightening. In women under distress, the monthly cycle becomes irregular or stops completely. In men, the sexual urge and the sperm cell formation are diminished.

A CASE OF DISTRESS

Susan married Robert at the age of 23. Their financial situation was typical of newlyweds: bad. Robert had just entered graduate school, and Susan was close to receiving her degree in education.

Susan soon finished school and found a teaching position in their small town. The money pinch eased somewhat, and the future looked brighter.

As they started their second year together, the routine of living was well established. Robert drove Susan to work and picked her up after his classes. They didn't have much leisure time together, what with Susan's preparation for teaching and Robert's studies.

Slowly Susan became aware she wasn't making Robert happy. He seemed to have raised his ideals of what his wife should be, and he let her know she wasn't rising with them. In loving him, she was willing to assume the blame and attempted to work out the problems that came between them.

Returning home early one day to pick up some papers, Susan walked into a classic shock situation. Robert was in the bedroom with another woman. Not knowing how to handle this, in her pain, she left without being noticed. Frantically she tried to analyze the situation from all angles, logical and hysterical. Finally she settled on the common approach, "pretend it isn't there and it will go away." It works very well as a mental time bomb. Perhaps you've tried it yourself? Distress in large doses appeared in Susan's life.

Susan and Robert planned to visit her parents over a long weekend. The day before they were to leave, Robert told her the car would have to go into the garage for five days and $160 worth of repairs. Giving Robert the money, she got on the train alone, having lost her hope of having time together to heal the rifts in their marriage.

When she returned, a faculty member at school asked her how she and Robert had done at the racetrack that weekend, and had she done something different to her hair? Susan immediately called the garage. Nothing had been wrong with her car.

Susan was approaching her capacity of patience and distress. She confronted Robert with her knowledge, remaining "reasonable and undramatic" in an effort to save a marriage that meant so much to her. She was willing to take half the blame and to forget his adventures. Robert knew that getting his degree in engineering would be difficult without Susan, and he was also aware of her need to make their marriage work. Agreeing to stop seeing other women was easy. Keeping the agreement was different.

Robert received his degree and accepted a job offer in Chicago. Susan feared cities, as Robert knew, but the opportunity was "unrefusable," he said.

A new apartment in the near north part of the city, a new job for Susan with a jealous, insecure principal, and her fear and dislike of the city added new layers of distress to her life. Susan remained cool, trying to deal with every situation by suppressing anxiety and carrying the responsibility.

Robert had many late business meetings (politics seemed to be a vital part of success). Rarely did he return home before midnight. On the day Susan again came home and heard sounds on the other side of the bedroom door, patience was finally forgotten. With distress at a frantic maximum, she left swearing never to come back. A teacher she worked with was the only person she could turn to in the strange city, with no money but lots of fear. The friend called me.

I came by and casually began talking with Susan. We talked the whole night. Susan, a sensitive and intelligent woman, was reasoning out her problems while she spoke. To prompt her to go on, I spoke of a woman with problems similar to hers and told Susan how she faced them. In comparing lives, Susan began to realize how tension, guilt, and fear—those roots of distress—affected her unnecessarily. I gave her Dr. Hans Selye's book, *The Stress of Life.* After reading it she decided to do something positive about her situation.

ANALYZING THE DISTRESS

Dividing the distress in Susan's life into two kinds, private and professional, we posed the following important questions for each category:

1. Can you handle it?
2. Do you have to handle it?
3. Can you change it?

All of these questions require courage and a lining up of priorities. In Susan's private life, tight finances, city living, Robert's criticisms, his infidelities, and the death of their love were her battles. Professionally, a tense relationship with a superior was something she felt she must endure if she could.

The next step was to find Susan's stress limit, the point where stress becomes distress. Recalling her various tension situations at home and at work, then analyzing them in terms of those limits, took a bit longer. When she found herself in control and able to handle distress, she had reached the turning point.

Being repeatedly rejected by her husband was a distress she didn't have to put up with. A relationship built on pain was harmful to her. She also decided not to take the additional, unnecessary distress of her jealous superior at work. She is now a single, successful business woman working for a large department store. Susan learned to analyze her distress and handle it.

Distress And Physical Damage

In prehistoric times, the situation was much simpler. Encountering danger, we decided either to run or to stand and fight. Our bodies prepared us for action by pouring adrenal hormones into our blood streams. Our hearts beat faster. The blood composition changed so that, in case of injury, it could clot faster. Blood vessels constricted, and the pumping of the heart raised our blood pressure.

When modern people are under distress, our bodies react much as they did in those of our primitive ancestors. But because our social structure allows us no outlet for the tensions which distress creates, we just sit there and grind our teeth. If distress situations occur frequently, the adrenal changes can bring on physical damage including inflammatory and atheriosclerotic changes in the blood vessels.

In handling modern stress, we must learn to find our limits and to keep tension at controllable levels. A basic knowledge of distress and how it ages you is a good starting point. Knowing your enemy is still the best way to win.

We pass through two basic stages when we are under distress. First, our bodies react with adrenal changes. Then, whether action is taken or not, we either adapt to the situation or the distress overcomes us and wears us down mentally and physically.

STRESS AND AGING

Stress, when it changes into distress, can render us vulnerable to many diseases that accelerate the rate of aging. A boss who gives you ulcers, a mate who irritates you, a traffic jam that makes you late for an important appointment, an impossible deadline: All these everyday distress situations can build up to take years off our lives.

In a recent seminar, air traffic controllers were singled out as people who are under immense distress. Being responsible for thousands of lives every minute has made these people excellent guinea pigs for stress research. Out of 111 air traffic controllers observed in a recent study, 86 showed signs of peptic ulcers, a classic distress symptom.

At the same meeting, the increasing incidence of cardiovascular disability among pilots was also demonstrated. While between 1953 and 1964 about 27 percent of pilots' disabilities were due to cardiovascular problems, in 1971 the proportion had increased to 44 percent. In that interval air traffic had increased in density, the airlines used larger and faster planes, and jets replaced the propeller. All these changes had also caused higher distress levels and a deterioration in the overall health of the pilots.

As a pilot, I am familiar with the habits of airline personnel; the irregular working hours and eating patterns are other contributing factors to their distress situation. If a pilot must get up at 3 A.M., seldom is breakfast available. At that hour blood sugar is low, and thinking is sluggish. Water soluble vitamins such as B and C have been flushed out of the system, and so the brain receives below-standard nutrients. A quick cup of coffee doesn't solve the problem. Dr. Carlton Fredericks recently reported that out of 177 pilots he studied, 40 suffered from hypoglycemia. These findings have taught us a lesson, and today pilots are given instruction about stress and the factors that contribute to changing it into distress.

THE STRESS TO WIN

Pilots are not the only ones who are under distress. In our daily lives, the obsession to win, to succeed, puts all of us under pressure, starting at the Little League level. Too often our schools place the emphasis on winning, not on trying. Professional sports teams are praised only if they win; the performance is of small consequence. Listen to the critics if two games are lost in a row!

We should learn to use sports as a release for distress, a way to relax, and not to multiply our tensions. This obsession to win is carried into every part of our daily lives, from having the cleanest house and car in the neighborhood, to being the "perfect" wife, or husband, or parent. Competition is good to the degree that it helps you to perform at your best level, but if overdoing it puts you on the psychiatrist's couch or the doctor's table, you should make some drastic revisions in your life.

SOME RECENT FINDINGS

Dr. Hans Selye of Canada, who has been working in the field of stress for a long time, recently discussed a new group of hormones that he calls catatoxic steroids. These hormones stimulate the formation of enzymes able to destroy the toxic substances that normally result from a stress situation. Smoking will introduce toxic materials into the blood stream, creating such a stress situation. If the catatoxic hormones function well, they detoxify our bodies by destroying nicotine and cancer-causing chemicals. Thus, there is evidence these hormones could protect us from cancer. However, there is a limit to their effectiveness. If a stress situation is too high—smoking more cigarettes than our body can handle, for example—the balance is shifted, true distress is the result, and the excess toxic materials go to work on your body. If at the same time cancer-causing chemicals are introduced into the body in foods, water, or air, the equilibrium is even further disturbed, and the risk of cancer increases.

In other studies, Dr. Selye was able to induce arthritis, ulcers, heart disease, and other disorders, by putting test animals under distress. What is even more interesting is the fact that the animals could be taught how to avoid stress situations. When these trained animals were subjected to stress, they avoided it and did not get ulcers; stress had not turned into distress. We can apply these lessons to humans.

Five Basic Steps In Coping With Distress

1. Learn what stress can do to you, how it ages you, and how it damages your health. Read Dr. Selye's *Stress Without Distress.*

2. Find your stress limits; recognize when stress changes into distress. Keep a record of distress symptoms such as a fast heartbeat, tense muscles, or a feeling in your stomach like a bundle of knots. Whenever you start grinding your teeth record that, too. Does this type of stress wear you out or do you thrive on it? How often do you go over your limit or come close to it? Are you exhausted after a few situations like this?

3. Evaluate your life in terms of distress. Analyze both your work situation and your private life. Keep adversity in perspective. Try to be rational about what is really important to

you. Make a change if necessary. If you are trying to go through a brick wall, the wall will win.

4. If you should become ill, speak with your doctor and make sure that he or she listens. Your physician should be familiar with your psychologically vulnerable points. Accept responsibility for your health. Don't expect your doctor to mend all that you have neglected. Accept the responsibility of helping him to heal you.

5. Finally, if your life seems too complex, try to simplify it. Avoid making adverse or unnecessary moves, but do not be afraid to alter situations that are detrimental to you and that can be changed. Keep an open mind about psychotherapy. The fewer mysteries your own psyche has for you, the lower your chances of suffering distress-related diseases.

The Ups and Downs in Our Lives

One morning a few years ago I found myself extremely irritable and physically exhausted for no apparent reason. A friend watched me for a while and commented, "Maybe your biorhythm curves are down."

"Sure," I replied, "and maybe the position of the moon has an effect on the protein content of the eggs I am eating!"

My friend was quite annoyed with my answer but proceeded to tell me about biorhythm curves. There are three major cycles a person goes through, she said, starting with the day of birth. It's as if your body goes through charge and discharge cycles.

The physical cycle is 23 days long. For the first 11 ½ days you are full of energy, your endurance is up, and you have reserves. In the second half of the cycle, another 11 ½ days, you are in the recharge period, and you shouldn't expect much from yourself.

The 28-day emotional cycle controls the nervous system.

111

During the first 14 days, you tend to be more optimistic, and your entire outlook on life is more positive. During the second half of the cycle, you are irritable because your emotional energy level is down.

The longest cycle is the intellectual cycle of 33 days, which reflects the functioning of your brain cells. During the first half of the cycle, 16 ½ days, you can learn and retain new information with higher capacity. In the second half of your intellectual cycle, the recharge period, it is better to review and work with the things you have learned.

Days when the cycles are changing from up to down or vice versa are considered critical, my friend told me. At such times we are likely to find life very turbulent. On these days we are also more accident prone. When you are at the highest or lowest point of a curve, this is considered a minicritical day.

A SCIENTIST'S ENCOUNTER WITH BIORHYTHM

As a trained scientist, I found it difficult to accept such ideas immediately. Remembering my former research advisor's advice, "give the impossible a chance," I decided that during the following months I would record daily my emotional highs and lows, my times of physical strength and weakness, my periods of mental inquisitiveness and dullness.

When I charted my findings, to my surprise approximately 80 percent of my good and bad days agreed with the predicted biorhythm curves. The projected critical days fit with more than 80 percent accuracy, and those that didn't agree were explainable by my diary. For example, on a day when my curves were up I was feeling well until three bad-news letters and a bent fender from a hit-and-run driver reversed my feelings. Another day my mood was up while my curves were down, according to my diary. On this day I had received a notice in the mail that one of my books had been accepted for publication. Of course, biorhythm calculations cannot predict outside influences.

All this was interesting but certainly not conclusive. I initiated a literature study that convinced me there was a great deal of validity in the theories of biorhythm and that we can better deal with the distress in our lives by becoming familiar with our biorhythm curves.

George Thommen, in his book *Is This Your Day?*, reports a number of telling examples of the influence of biorhythms. Scott Carpenter, the astronaut, overshot his landing 250 miles on May 24, 1962, when he was near a critical day in his sensitivity curve and his physical curve was low. An airline pilot crashed, for no apparent reason, when his biorhythm curves were critical. Arnold Palmer won a golf tournament in England when all his biorhythm curves were up, and lost the PGA two weeks later when all his curves were down.

Statistics in many countries indicate that biorhythm has its place among the sciences. To improve the exchange of ideas among researchers in this field, the International Biorhythm Research Association (IBRA) was founded in July 1977; its offices are located in Atlanta.

RESEARCH FINDINGS ABOUT BIORHYTHM

In Japan the entire transportation industry is based on biorhythm. From airline pilots to bus drivers, workers are alerted to their critical times and, in many cases, given those days off. Accident rates were reduced tremendously, more than 60 percent in some studies. In Switzerland, a team of doctors found that more than six times as many heart attacks and strokes occurred on critical days and that postoperative death rates were higher when operations were performed on patients' critical days. In Germany, it was found that normally good students who flunked exams had taken them on a critical day. In another study it was found that personal injuries were 85 percent more likely to occur on critical days.

In the United States, research teams successfully predicted the outcome of sports events by using biorhythm. Much of this material is presented in *Biorhythm Sports Forecasting* by Bernard Gittelson, who also wrote a superb introductory book on biorhythm called *Biorhythm, A Personal Science* (Arco). In Denver, a cab company advised its drivers of critical biorhythm days and reduced its accident rate by 50 percent. Several U.S. airlines advise their flight crews on biorhythms, and the results available thus far are very convincing.

In one of my own studies, I found that people were able to lose weight more easily if they were advised on biorhythm.

During the founding meeting of IBRA in Atlanta, Walter Appel from Germany and Professor Sigmund Kardas, presently teaching in Spain, reported that conductivity measurements on the skin of humans confirmed the existence of biorhythm curves.

USING BIORHYTHM TO COMBAT DISTRESS

Biorhythm calculations are rather complicated and until recently were made only by experts. Now the computations have been simplified through the use of slide rules and calculators that allow you to calculate the positions of your curves. The most sophisticated of these devices is an electronic calculator called Kosmos 1. This machine lets you know, by means of red and yellow lights, when you have critical or minicritical days. It displays the positions of your biorhythm curves if you merely punch in your birth date and the present date. Since it also has a memory, you can calculate the biorhythmic compatibility between yourself and another person.

Many people have discovered that by learning about their biorhythm curves, they are in a better position to deal with stressful situations. Biorhythm can help prevent the stress of a situation from becoming distress. Knowing the days when you have extra reserves, or when you shouldn't expect too much from yourself because your curves are down, can smooth out an otherwise highly stressful day. When you know you will have a double critical on an important day, it might even be better to "put off until tomorrow" a difficult task or painful decision.

Since no one has yet been able to show exactly why biorhythm works, I was at first reluctant to include it in the Multi-Factorial Approach to better health. But the statistics and my own experiences convinced me: Biorhythm should be an important part of any serious program to fight stress and slow down the aging process.

Chapter 9

Buying Time

"Our present retirement system can lead to physical and emotional illness and premature death."

A statement by the American Medical Association, 1974.

The Money Quiz	*Yes*	*No*

1. Are you 100 percent sure that, after retirement or in an emergency, you don't have to rely solely on social security? — —
2. Do you have an investment program, or savings, to assure yourself reasonable financial independence after retirement or in an emergency? — —
3. Is a retirement income from your place of work a certainty, and do you know how much you will get? — —
4. Do you know that your income after retirement will meet your needs? — —
5. Do you have enough insurance coverage so

116

that an extended illness or hospital stay
won't cause a financial disaster? — —
6. Are the other members of your family
reasonably well protected financially? — —
7. Do you have a financial reserve so that you
could live for two months without any
income? — —

If you answered all questions "yes," move on to the next
chapter.

If you answered 2, 3, and 5 "yes" but missed some of the
other questions, you might move on but come back to this
chapter later.

If you answered more than four questions "no," read this
chapter carefully.

When I speak about aging to social clubs, business organizations, and groups of college students, I frequently ask people in the audience which factors they think contribute to
living a happier and longer life. Some of the most common
answers include long walks, good nutrition, clean air, heredity, deep breathing exercises, yoga, ginseng, no smoking,
drinking only wine and no strong alcoholic drinks, swimming
half an hour every day, having a good nature, and being
relaxed and without stress. But nobody ever says "money."
Quite frankly, I never considered it a life-extending force
either until I started interviewing older people who lived in
inexpensive retirement homes.

When I asked them, "Why don't you have a reasonable
amount of money to spend?", I heard the same answers over
and over again.

"I thought I would get a good retirement check from my
company."

"I was paying so much money into social security, I thought

I would get a good retirement from it."

"I changed jobs and lost my retirement benefits."

"I never thought about retirement until it was about to happen."

"I didn't really know how much money I could have saved if I had put a few dollars into a retirement program."

"Who wants to think about retirement when you're young? I had such a good time spending my money, I couldn't have cared less what would happen when I got older."

Of course, it's not just our senior citizens whose activities are curtailed by a shortage of funds. But for most younger people, the money factor is not so much a question of having enough as of using it wisely. We all know that the best things in life cannot be bought. But money *is* a factor in longevity, whether you think in terms of material comfort, medical care, the standard of living, or being able to afford a "revitalization" vacation in Europe.

Most of the measures recommended in this book for prolonging your lifespan are not expensive; in fact, many of them can save you money, either immediately (how much could you save by giving up smoking?) or in the long run by preventing expensive illnesses. Our society must take the blame for the fact that so many senior citizens, who could still lead vigorous lives, must bear the double burdens of poverty and inactivity. But there is much that we can do while still young to improve our attitudes toward money so we can retire with financial security.

Money-Saving Health Tips

Depending on your age, marital status, and where you live, there are quite a few areas of spending that you could probably cut down on easily. The ones most of us have in common are junk foods, soft drinks, and cigarettes: all unnecessary; all expensive; all bad for you. If you think carefully about your life style, you can probably come up with several others. Naturally, there are people who are financially independent so that, no matter what they do and spend, they'll always have sufficient backing. However, many of us are not so lucky. If saving a few dollars here and there, without putting major limitations on our life style, will make the difference between security after retirement and having to live in a low-income retirement home (very saddening institutions), we should start to think and act reasonably. The paragraphs below suggest some other ways to save money.

When you are out for an evening, that one drink too many —the one you don't finish, or the one you wish you hadn't had —is an avoidable expense. Also, how about buying a less costly drink? A nonalcoholic drink if you are just thirsty, or beer or wine instead of scotch or bourbon? If you don't think you could save $2 or 3 per day this way, just look around you and observe what the person next to you is spending on drinks.

Do you often feel the urge for a sweet treat? Try eating fruit instead. Take an apple to work for your midmorning snack rather than buying a doughnut.

How much do you spend each week on candy, a quick coke, an over-priced snack in a movie theater, etc.? Remember how these expenses add up. The impact will hit you in the wallet as well as the waistline.

Do you often drive somewhere when you could have walked the short distance? The cost of operating a car is highest when short distances are involved.

Never do your food shopping before a meal or when you are very hungry! Wait until after the meal or eat something first; otherwise you'll waste a lot of money on unnecessary food items.

Most good restaurants are expensive, but they serve you a lot of delicious foods for the money you pay. We often feel that, since we paid for it and since it tastes so good, we shouldn't let anything go to waste and so we stuff ourselves. Afterwards, we aren't good for anything else for at least a few hours, and if we make a habit of this, we might get fat. A man in Chicago came to see me once, because things "just weren't as they used to be." After a usually exhausting day at the office, he would take his dates to a show, then to an expensive restaurant for a big meal and drinks, and then home to his apartment. And that's where, in many ways, the trouble started. He had no idea that a man's sexual performance, among other things, was strongly affected by his life style and physiology. So, why not ask your date to share an entree with you? Eat early in the evening rather than immediately before you go to bed. Maybe order just an extra salad. The overall results will be that you'll save about $10 per evening, you'll be peppier, and you will not have risked your health.

Over-the-counter drugs and other drugstore items are often health risks, due to their side effects, and a waste of money. If aspirin was discovered today, it would never make it on the shelves as a nonprescription drug because its side effects are so numerous. Yet most Americans, from junior-high-school students to the most well-educated adults, reach unthinkingly for the aspirin whenever they have the slightest headache. Do you think you need a laxative? Try increasing the roughage in your diet instead. A mouthwash? Brush your teeth. Drugs to calm your stomach? They can ruin your intestinal acid balance and hide signs of true disorders. A new lipstick or fingernail polish? Have you used up any one of the last 20 you bought? The list could continue.

The savings possible in the areas mentioned above could average at least $5 a day. At the same time, you could also lose some weight, decrease your health risks, put less stress on your liver, lower your chance of becoming an alcoholic, decrease your cancer and heart disease risk, and age at a slower rate.

INTEREST RATES

There are numerous other ways to save money. Do you ever take out high-interest loans? That's usually what you're in for when you purchase something with little or no down payment. Charge accounts and credit cards, if carelessly used, can be a tremendous waste of money. For the small privilege of being able to get things exactly when we want them, we often pay for the rest of our lives if we are not careful.

I recently asked some friends who had credit cards to tell me the monthly balances on which they paid interest. Their answers ranged from $500 to 5,000. At the usual interest rate of 18 percent per year, they were paying from $90 to 900 per year for their privileges.

If they had not burdened themselves with that kind of debt, their money could instead be working for them. In order to determine the interest rate on which to base long-term calculations (20 to 40 years into the future), I consulted some financial experts and got some interesting advice. Most savings banks pay 5 ¾ to 7 ¾ percent interest which, when compounded monthly, is an effective 6 to 8 percent. There are numerous 8 percent tax-free bond issues available. Some other bonds are taxed only when you sell them; if you keep them until you retire, your taxes will be low. On larger amounts of money ($50,000 and up) one can get interest rates of up to 9 ¼ percent. In the past few decades interest rates have gone up an average of ½ percent every 6 to 9 years; they sometimes leveled off, but rarely went down. On that basis, my advisers suggested that we could base long-term calculations on a 9 ½ percent interest rate. Since in some cases taxes will have to be paid, it is more reasonable to assume that you can earn 7 ½ percent to 8 percent interest. These rates might be available only for larger sums of money, in which case daily savings could be banked at a lower interest rate until enough had built up to qualify for the higher return. Ask your bank's personal finance consultant for more information.

Let's see how much money you could accrue by investing an average daily saving of $5 to $10 over a longer time period.

How much could you save per day if you really tried?

Now let's see how much my friends could have accrued if they had invested the money they spent on finance charges.

How much interest are you paying on your charge accounts and credit cards?

Money saved per day and invested in a 7½% interest account	Total accrued money after		
	10 years	20 years	30 years
$5 per day ($1,825 per year)	$25,805	$ 78,475	$187,975
$10 per day ($3,650 per year)	$51,610	$156,950	$375,950

Monthly balance on which they paid interest	Annual finance charge they incurred	Amount they would have accrued by investing the finance charge at 7.5% after		
		10 years	20 years	30 years
$ 500	$ 90	$ 1,272	$ 3,870	$ 9,270
$1,000	$180	$ 2,545	$ 7,740	$18,540
$2,000	$360	$ 5,090	$15,480	$37,080
$3,000	$540	$ 7,635	$23,220	$55,620
$4,000	$720	$10,180	$30,960	$74,160
$5,000	$900	$12,726	$38,700	$92,700

Use your charge accounts only when absolutely necessary, and only when you *know* how you are going to pay for them. Pay them off as soon as possible; they are serving you well only if you pay your bills before you are charged interest.

Social Security: The Big Rip-Off?

Why am I placing so much emphasis on developing your own savings or investment plan? The answer is that you just can't count on social security income to give you a comfortable standard of living after retirement. Actually, taking inflation rates and projected social security payments into account, only one thing is certain: Despite all the money you paid into this system, it will not enable you to live above sub-subpoverty levels.

Economist Peter Somers of the University of California has called social security "the biggest single roadblock to the security of the American wage earner." An Illinois insurance executive has said, "If a private insurance company attempted to sell a plan in Illinois which cost so much and paid so little, we would drum them out of the state as frauds." And backing up the experts' opinions are the thousands of elderly people subsisting on the poverty-level income of so-called social security "benefits."

THE TROUBLE WITH SOCIAL SECURITY

Critics of our present system of social security—and these include many of our most concerned political leaders, business executives, and private citizens—point out that it discriminates against many people, that there are many abuses, and that the money paid into the system is spent immediately so that it can't carry any interest for you. But the main problem with social security is that the returns on your money, compared to what you could get on the open money market, are so incredibly low.

As an example, let's take a case the Social Security Administration uses in one of its brochures. The year is 1974; a hypothetical 40-year-old worker expects to retire in 1999 at the age of 65. Between now and retirement, the worker will have contributed $41,839 to the social security system. At retirement, the "potential benefit" available to this worker is $128,618.

That may sound impressive, but it isn't. The social security system actually receives *twice* the $41,839 paid by the employee, since the employer must match the employee's contributions. So a more accurate figure for the total payment to social security necessary to obtain that "potential benefit" is $83,678, or an average of $3,347 a year. If this annual deduction were invested at 8 percent interest, instead of being given to the Social Security Administration, the worker would have accumulated a $244,685 nest egg by the time of retirement. This is nearly twice the "potential benefit" offered by social security. If we assume a 7 percent interest rate, the account balance at retirement would be $211,694; still almost two-thirds more than social security offers as a "potential benefit."

The figures for a 22-year-old worker are even more stunning. In return for payments totaling $233,598 by the time the worker turns 65, the Social Security Administration offers a "potential benefit" of $329,556. At 8 percent interest, the same annual payments would have built a nest egg of $1,790,278 at the worker's 65th birthday; at 7 percent interest the equivalent figure would be $1,345,920.

These examples are intended only to demonstrate the magnitude of the waste, and the figures for any individual will vary. I am not implying that we should all build up such huge amounts of money in personal savings accounts, since experts on the subject say this could hurt the economy.

TOWARD A MORE HONEST SYSTEM

A better, more effective system of social security is a must; that's the one thing the experts agree on. Numerous suggestions have been made. Perhaps the best approach would be to make it mandatory for each individual to build a personal system of financial security at a place of his or her own choice, at a bank, an insurance company, or even by buying social security bonds. The employer would make payments into the retirement account at set time intervals. Even allowing for the fact that the change-over to a new system always costs money, the overall return, carrying some of the change-over costs ourselves, would be many times what it is now.

If the actual buildup of money in security accounts does not appear desirable, we could establish a point system. Our payments into the security account at banks, insurance companies, or the new social security administration would "buy" credit points worth a certain monthly allowance at retirement, a set number of weekly disability payments, or a specific amount of medical insurance coverage.

To help pay for the new system, we could eliminate waste, mismanagement, fraud, and duplication in existing social programs.

Some Needed Changes in Attitude

The need for many reforms in our present systems should be crystal clear by now. But that kind of social reform must also be accompanied by wide-reaching changes in our attitude toward retirement.

We all know examples of people who led active lives until they were forced to retire because of age. Too often, people who have worked all their lives find it impossible to deal with vast stretches of empty time. They become depressed, irrita-

125

ble, and sickly, a burden on their families and their communities.

This kind of situation need not be common. Retirement can be rewarding if people know how to cope with increased leisure time and are prepared for it both psychologically and economically.

American business is caught up in the youth culture of our times. It has a tendency to pamper young, relatively low-cost employees in the mistaken belief that they are more productive and imaginative. Older workers often get pushed into doing routine work which they don't really enjoy, but they accept the situation in the belief that they can't hope for anything better.

Today many people are staying active longer and are willing to work longer to improve their retirement benefits. What is more important, they are capable of doing it. To set the retirement age arbitrarily at 65 just doesn't make sense in light of what we know about the human capacity for work and learning. Older people, especially when they are *willing* to learn, can adapt themselves to new situations. They can be retrained and they can go back to school at any age. Instead of setting a retirement age at 65, we should evaluate employees by their capacity and willingness to handle present or new jobs.

One important way in which we could improve our present system would be to soften the transition between full-time employment and complete retirement. As retirement approaches, we should give employees increasing amounts of time off so that they get used to their leisure. In England, some unions are already pressing for extended vacation time in the last years before retirement. Earlier and more extensive financial planning is also essential to a rewarding retirement. Labor pacts recently signed by certain container industries and branches of the aluminum industry provide retirement

packages which, with social security, will give pensions totaling up to 85 percent of employees' salaries.

Retirement counseling and planning should start no later
than the age of 40 (and some experts say our high schools
should offer courses on the subject). People should be made
aware of the financial choices they will have; they should be
educated about how much money they can expect, how much
they should save, and the options available to them.

Where and under what conditions to retire is another question very few people seriously consider. If you live in an ugly,
polluted environment, it will have a dramatic effect on your
overall health. Can you afford to sell your home and move
somewhere else? Is your present environment good for your
health? Do you have serious ragweed allergies? Don't retire
in the Midwest. Does altitude bother your breathing? Don't
retire in the mountains. Are you planning to move into a
retirement home? Think carefully. It may be unnatural for
you to move out of your usual varied environment and into
an atmosphere in which everyone is similar to you in age and
outlook.

Planning for retirement is essential if later years are to be
livable. By the time you reach retirement age, you *can* be
physically fit, have a reasonable amount of money, and know
how to fill your leisure time. When you finally retire under
these conditions, the world is open for you and you can enjoy
many of the activities you have always hoped that retirement
would allow. You *can* plan your own future.

If the numbers cited in this chapter aren't enough to encourage you to start your own retirement planning, consider
the conditions you might have to live under if you don't have
a reasonable amount of money after retirement. Ever visit a
low-cost retirement home? How would you live on a social
security income of $160 or even $360 per month?

127

What About Retirement Homes?

If you are already retired, you may be considering moving to a retirement home. If so, you should remember one very important life-prolonging measure: *Stay out of a retirement home.*

It is my view that taking people out of their natural environment as they get older, and putting them into retirement homes, is a cruel and irresponsible thing to do. No matter how gilded the cage might be, there is nothing to be gained from such an approach. Mary Adelaide Mendelson, in her book *Tender Loving Greed,* says: "Behind the thievery and the corruption that this book describes is the physical reality of the stinking nursing homes in which our old people are dying a living death."

When Dr. Neil Solomon, Maryland's Secretary of Mental Health and Hygiene, was asked his advice about nursing homes recently, he said: "Let me emphasize as strongly as possible that we always advocate, whenever possible, a noninstitutional arrangement in preference to a nursing home or other institution." To foster such noninstitutional alternatives, Maryland has instituted a system through which physicians, nurses, and social workers visit the elderly in their homes. Telephone answering services keep social aid people in touch with seniors. Older people have the help they need without losing touch with the larger society. Maryland's plan is a step in the right direction, and similar programs have been started in other states.

Long before you retire you should remember one piece of advice: no matter how, when, or where you retire, the important thing is to plan ahead so you will have enough money to make your senior years pleasant and free of worry.

Part III

Fighting the Most Serious Causes of Aging

A person who reaches age 45 today can expect to live only three years longer than a person who reached 45 in 1900.

Chapter 10

The Case for Prevention

"Those who have lived the longest seem to be those remote from medical practice, as well as other aspects of modern civilization."

Ruth B. Weg, Ph.D., in
Aging: Prospects and Issues

The most important steps we can take toward living a longer and more active life are those that have been shown to help prevent accidents and diseases. As Professor B. L. Strehler of the University of Southern California told the American Association for the Advancement of Science in 1974, any illness or injury is a contributing factor to aging and, if prevented, can slow down the entire process of growing old.

The degree to which a sickness contributes to overall aging depends very much on the type of disease, its frequency, and the susceptibility of the individual. Diseases also limit our ability to exercise and thus prevent us from staying fit.

Many people take a rather carefree attitude toward prevention in their belief that modern medicine can cure virtually anything. Not so! No matter how optimistic the latest discoveries might sound, the survival rate for victims of most major diseases is extremely low. In the treatment of lung cancer, even with early detection and surgery, only about 7 percent of patients survive for five years. In people with severe heart disease, 21 percent of heart bypass operations become ineffective within five months. And there is no real treatment for heart attacks or for blood clots in the brain; if the victim survives an attack or stroke, his doctor can only hope to make him feel comfortable. All the efforts of our medical and scientific experts can't rectify the serious problems that result from years of poor health habits.

One of the major reasons for emphasizing the importance of prevention—and this is of special urgency for people above 50—is that some diseases can be prevented but not cured. The most notable are heart attacks and cancer. Of course, these are not the only diseases which can be prevented, but since they are the predominant causes of death in this country (about 75 percent of the people who die each year are killed by heart trouble and cancer), it seems worthwhile to take special precautions against them. Such a program is discussed in the next two chapters.

If diseases are not prevented and drugs are used in treatment, their side effects can be detrimental to our health and longevity. Should the problem be life-threatening (cancer, for example), we often have to use drug levels so high that only time can tell whether the drug will wipe out the disease before it kills the patient. Even in the treatment of less serious illnesses, Americans often use drugs unnecessarily, or in needlessly high amounts. The aspirin you take for your headache can have severe negative side-effects. Preventing the headache in the first place, perhaps by analyzing and coping with tension in a new way, is the safest policy. And the same thinking should be applied before we take any prescription or over-the-counter medication.

One of the most important health factors to which prevention can be applied is stress. According to Dr. Hans Selye, any disease causes distress; and any distress situation can also bring on disease. When we are under undue pressure, we don't function well; our endocrine system is affected, our sex life suffers, and we become susceptible to things that are harmless under normal conditions. The result: an accelerated rate of aging.

Prevention can also protect us from the many diseases that affect the immune system, our first line of defense against toxic materials and harmful bacteria and viruses. Any disease that affects the thymus, blood-cell formation, or the functioning of the bone marrow, belongs in this category. People with a malfunctioning immune system have an accelerated rate of aging and a shorter lifespan.

Evidence is mounting that several diseases, including some old-age afflictions, can originate with faulty nutrition in the prenatal period. The susceptibility to diabetes, which is largely hereditary, and several diseases of the arteries, can be controlled by an early preventive approach.

As explained earlier, a substantial and well-trained amount of muscle tissue is one of the best safeguards against disorders associated with glucose metabolism. Thus a sensible program of prevention is our best weapon against hypoglycemia and diabetes. Likewise, the earliest possible practice of preventive measures is important for the avoidance of senility and mental disorders.

So far I have mentioned several arguments for prevention, and there are many more. Throughout this book, you will see more examples of the crucial role prevention plays in other areas of health and aging, from a headache to a cold, from heart attacks and cancer to VD.

And speaking of venereal disease, this is an area in which prevention is crucially needed. The spread of social diseases could be dramatically decreased if everybody would take basic precautions and be honest with their sexual partners about the subject. Even in our "liberated" times, too often carriers do not inform others with whom they have had intercourse of the problem. Douching, cleanliness, and washing help prevent VD, but regular blood tests for syphilis and a simple smear test for gonorrhea should be parts of all our lives. A man will know when he has gonorrhea, but a woman will find it difficult to detect.

The best suggestion I have heard so far for dealing with our vast VD problem came from Dr. David Reuben, who suggested a VD day or week during which everybody would go to a doctor or clinic and have a VD check. Such a program would virtually eliminate VD in the United States. But until our society takes such steps, each of us must seek tests individually as part of an overall prevention program. Wouldn't you like the idea that others are as careful as you and would notify you immediately if any problem existed?

The need for a stronger emphasis on prevention is established through health and survival statistics. While the United States spends more money on medical care than any other country, in terms of overall health and average lifespan America ranks twentieth. Also, a person who reaches age 45 today can expect to live only about three years longer than a person who had reached age 45 in 1900.

Where Can You Get Preventive Care?

You can get preventive health care from your doctor and local hospital (you should be covered by insurance), and the health maintenance organizations (HMOs) have taken some promising steps in this direction. If you belong to an HMO, you pay a certain premium per year for health care to keep you well. Unnecessary medication and hospitalization are therefore greatly reduced.

This basic idea of the HMO is good, but many doctors in HMOs are not yet convinced that diseases can be prevented, and that the preventive approach is less expensive although both facts are well documented in medical literature.

I have designed several computer programs to help doctors teach their patients the importance of nutrition and good health habits, but our medical professionals are not comfortable with new ideas. However, those who have come over to the preventive approach never go back to their previous methods. And patients, asking their doctors questions about nutrition, have been very helpful in getting them to explore the preventive approach.

To find a prevention-oriented doctor in your area, you can write to any one of the following organizations. Your letter should be short (don't enclose your medical history); just tell where you live and ask for a list of member doctors in your area. Please enclose whatever donation you can afford; these are nonprofit organizations.

International Academy of Preventive Medicine
10409 Town & Country Way, Suite 200
Houston, Texas 77024

International College of Applied Nutrition
P.O. Box 386
La Habra, Cal. 90631

The Academy of Orthomolecular Psychiatry
1691 Northern Blvd.
Manhasset, N.Y. 11030

True preventive care is also practiced by the American Prevention Institute (1425 Engracia Avenue, Torrance, Cal. 90501), where patients not only receive the correct treatments for the prevention of heart and other diseases, but they are also taught how to continue the preventive approach when they return to their normal environments.

Chapter 11

Preventing Heart Attacks

"No one has ever shown that eating cholesterol causes heart disease. If anyone can step forward and prove that eating cholesterol causes heart disease, I will donate all my proceeds from this book to the American Heart Association."

Richard Passwater, Ph.D.,
in *Supernutrition for Healthy Hearts*

Diseases of the circulatory system, leading to heart attacks, are America's number one killer, accounting for 50 percent of the nation's deaths each year. Once the heart becomes damaged, medicine can do little to repair it. But research indicates that circulatory problems can be averted by the proper preventive approach.

The results of recent experiments have made it possible to evaluate in detail the primary factors that contribute to diseases of the heart and arteries. My approach, as you will see, is quite different from that used by most doctors in this field, who have achieved little with their cholesterol- and triglyceride-lowering drugs, their blood pressure-regulating medications, and low cholesterol diets. During the 1976 spring meeting of the International Academy of Preventive Medicine, Nathan Pritikin, author of *Live Longer Now,* discussed the ineffectiveness of several conventional methods. He cited a five-year study of 8,000 men which evaluated the drugs given to coronary patients. The study indicated that the patients would have been better off if they had taken placebos.

Longevity studies with several types of animals have repeatedly shown that there are many different causes of aging and that, by interfering with several causes at the same time, we can extend life longer than by interfering with a single factor. Shouldn't the same thinking apply to diseases of the heart and arteries?

We know several things that contribute to circulatory disease. Each one makes some sense, but no single factor can explain everything. For a fuller picture we must consider a combination of the many causative elements.

What Is Coronary Heart Disease (CHD)?

The two major diseases of the arteries that lead to heart disease are atherosclerosis and arteriosclerosis. Atherosclerosis is a process in which narrowing of the arteries occurs. Several types of compounds (fats, cholesterol, proteins, minerals, etc.) are deposited on, and in, the arterial walls, thus limiting the flow of blood through the vessels. Once an artery is narrowed by such deposits, it is likely that more material will accumulate at the same spot. If the radius of an artery is reduced by one half, the blood flow is reduced to about one-sixteenth. Naturally, if the blood flow is constricted, this impairs the supply of nutrients to the various tissues.

There are several types of atherosclerosis, depending on where the narrowing of the arteries occurs. Angina pectoris, for example, is the narrowing of the arteries that link the heart

137

with the lungs. Thrombosis is the blocking of arteries, and again there are subdivisions like coronary thrombosis (leading to heart attacks) and cerebral thrombosis (leading to stroke).

Arteriosclerosis is the process in which arteries lose their elasticity. If the heart of a person with this disease starts pumping faster because of increased physical activity or a sudden emotion, his or her blood pressure increases tremendously. A rupture in a hardened artery is now more likely to occur. We must keep in mind, however, that high blood pressure itself does not harden the arteries.

Whether we are talking about atherosclerosis or arteriosclerosis, a limited blood flow is the result, and the final damage usually occurs after a blood clot forms and blocks an artery. When the blood flow is thus severely limited or completely closed off, other arteries must take over and supply blood via alternate pathways, if possible. Sometimes this is not possible, and the blood, with its nutrients and oxygen, cannot reach its destination. The fact that brain and heart cells have a lower storage capacity and must constantly be bathed in nutrient fluids makes this situation extremely serious. Even the most conservative nutritionists agree that an optimum supply of nutrients and oxygen is not achieved by a breakfast of doughnuts and coffee and a lunch of a ham sandwich on white bread with a Coke, topped off by smoking a pack of cigarettes a day.

The Causes of Diseases of the Arteries

In their attempts to find the causes of diseases of the arteries, researchers have discovered several possible culprits. Each time a new one is identified, they think they have solved the problem, until somebody else shows that the opposite of their findings can also be true. Some researchers argue for, and some against, cholesterol-containing foods; some are for and others against polyunsaturates; and each one has a set of studies to support his or her views. Why are we getting such confusing results in the heart studies?

The answer is simple: None of the studies carried out in the past has concentrated on good nutrition in combination with good health habits; only recently two such studies, still very incomplete, have pointed us in the right direction. Besides this, many of the studies follow the conventional approach of assuming that for every disease there must be a drug cure; this just isn't so in the case of heart disease. Furthermore, it is clear that the top five coronary heart disease risk factors are faulty nutrition, the lack of vitamins and minerals, being overweight, the lack of exercise, and smoking cigarettes.

Let's take a close look at what is known about the causes of heart disease.

CHOLESTEROL

Because cholesterol has been so much in the news in recent years, many people are already aware of what is called the cholesterol feedback mechanism. Our bodies have their own ways to synthesize cholesterol, and this process is slowed down if the blood cholesterol level is increased by the cholesterol in the foods we eat.

Drs. Joseph Goldstein and Michael Brown of the University of Texas Southwestern Medical School examined the tendency to accumulate cholesterol in the body and found that people who have this inherited disease have a defective cholesterol feedback mechanism.

According to Jeremiah Stamler, professor of community health and preventive medicine at Northwestern University in Chicago, the lowest rate of sudden death and all CHD deaths occur when cholesterol levels are around 200 milligrams per 100 milliliters of blood, abbreviated as 200 mg percent (a safe cut-off level was believed to be 220 mg percent). A report in the *Journal of the American Medical Association* stated that only about 20 percent of heart patients have serum cholesterol levels above 220, and newer research results suggest that levels in the range of 190 to 160, or even lower, are desirable.

Although the margarine industry would like us to believe that eating margarine rather than butter can help us keep cholesterol levels down and reduce our CHD risk, there is no evidence for such a claim. If this were true, we should have seen a decrease in the incidence of heart attacks in the past few years, because in that period margarine consumption has increased by 30 percent. But instead of decreasing, the number of heart attack victims—particularly women—has grown.

There is also no evidence to support claims made by some doctors that the amount of cholesterol in your diet has an effect on blood cholesterol levels. Several university studies repeatedly showed that increased cholesterol intakes, as high as the equivalent of 13 eggs per day, had no effect on blood cholesterol levels. For a detailed discussion of the contributing factors to CHD, read *Supernutrition for Healthy Hearts* by Richard Passwater (Dial Press); this is an excellent book and is also highly recommended to doctors working in this field.

Until proof is available to the contrary, we should consider blood cholesterol a possible cause of heart disease. Ask your doctor to analyze your cholesterol level at your next checkup, and to help you keep that level in the healthy range (but, please, without drugs).

Controlling Cholesterol Levels

In case cholesterol should turn out to be a contributing factor to heart disease, our main concern should be to prevent it from building up in and on the arteries. Emil Ginter of the Institute of Human Nutrition Research in Bratislava, Czechoslovakia, reported that vitamin C helps control the level of cholesterol by converting it into bile acid. Professor Ralph Mumma, of the University of Pennsylvania, showed that vitamin C and its derivatives can increase cholesterol excretion.

Another way to reduce blood cholesterol levels, or prevent an increase, is to exercise. A Harvard study of medical students, performed by Dr. George Mann, revealed that the subjects' cholesterol levels did not rise if they went on a high calorie diet and at the same time increased their physical activity, but that cholesterol levels did go up when subjects didn't exercise and when their weight increased.

The body needs cholesterol to make vitamin D and the sex and adrenocortical hormones. Since it is found together with fats, it is often classified as one even though this is chemically not correct. Fats, cholesterol, and many other compounds like phospholipids, lipoproteins, and steroids are all part of the large, operational (rather than structural) group of lipids.

An excessive intake of calories will increase the amount of fats (the chemical term is "triglycerides") in the blood, and since cholesterol is soluble in fat, it too will rise in most cases. Exercise will burn up (and therefore lower) the triglycerides, and cholesterol will also decrease.

Cholesterol is actually carried by two substances in the blood: low-density lipoprotein (LDL) takes it into the arteries, while high-density lipoprotein (HDL) gets rid of it. So, we would like a low LDL and a high HDL.

Dr. Peter D. Wood and his colleagues at the Stanford Heart Disease Prevention Program compared the ratios of these two compounds in middle-aged runners and in nonrunners. They found that exercise normalized the ratio, decreasing LDL and increasing HDL. The runners had half the triglyceride levels

141

of the nonrunners and HDL levels over 50 percent higher than the nonrunners.

Dr. Charles Glueck reported in *Atherosclerosis* (a MEDCOM publication) that the average plasma cholesterol level in American children ranges anywhere from 50 to 100 mg percent higher than levels in children from less-developed countries. I suggest that we take a new look at low-cholesterol baby foods as a possible cause of this problem. A breast-fed child gets a good deal of cholesterol from its mother, and this is the way nature intended it. If, on the other hand, a child is given foods with a low cholesterol content, its body has to make cholesterol to maintain a normal level in the blood. This forced increase in cholesterol synthesis among children might well lead to elevated cholesterol levels in their later years.

TRIGLYCERIDES

The amount of fat in the blood (the triglyceride level) appears to be a true indicator of atherosclerosis. Even though a 100 percent connection is not established, a cause-and-effect relationship is widely accepted among the experts.

Dr. J. Barboriak at Yale has demonstrated that it is entirely possible for animals to be fat yet not have atherosclerosis if, in addition to large amounts of fat, they are fed quality proteins, vitamins, and minerals. However, if the protein source is not the best, and if vitamins are not present in the diet in sufficient quantities, animals tend to develop atherosclerosis. Other studies indicate that vitamin B_6 is particularly important in a high fat diet. (An important tip for the person who eats a lot of junk foods.)

Changing from a diet high in saturated fat to one high in polyunsaturated fat does not lower triglyceride levels. It may even increase your risk of getting cancer. Such a diet also keeps triglycerides higher for a longer time than saturated fats do. High triglycerides can cause red blood cells to clump together and thus reduce the oxygen-carrying capacity of the blood.

Like the cholesterol level, the triglyceride level of your blood should be monitored closely by your doctor. Current studies indicate that triglyceride levels of about 100 or lower are desirable.

VITAMINS AND THE BLOOD

Several researchers have reported that vitamins C and E can reduce blood platelet adhesion—a very important discovery, since blood clotting is the cause of many heart attacks. British and Swedish scientists have reported that vitamin C does this by reducing the stickiness of the blood. These findings have forced many medical authorities, including some who were skeptical of vitamin therapy, to take a new look at the subject.

Vitamin B-15 (also known as gluconic 15, pangamic acid, and calcium pangamate) is a compound that increases the oxygen-carrying capacity of the blood. For a summary of recent findings regarding it, see Richard Passwater's articles in *Let's Live*, January and February 1976.

THE ROLE OF MINERALS

I have already discussed the importance of minerals, but there is one—calcium—that seems to play an especially important role in diseases of the heart and arteries. Dr. Margaret D. Crawford and her associates at the London School of Hygiene and Tropical Medicine examined the possible link be-

143

tween soft water and heart attacks by studying people from two towns, one with soft water, the other with hard water. They found that people from the soft-water town had more cholesterol in their systems and higher blood pressure than people in the hard-water town.

On the basis of several experiments, Professor Leo Lutwak of the University of California, Los Angeles, has concluded that we need about 1,000 to 1,200 milligrams of calcium per day, and that the ideal ratio of calcium to phosphorus in our food is about 1:1. According to an earlier study, our average daily calcium intake is about 400 milligrams per day, and the usual calcium-to-phosphorus ratio is about 1:2.5.

What happens if we deviate from the desirable calcium/-phosphorus ratio by increasing the phosphorus or decreasing the calcium? Experiments with animals show that such variations lead to secondary hyperparathyroidism, a disease in which abnormally high activity of the thyroid gland causes demineralization of bone and loss of calcium, ultimately leading to pain in the muscles.

Milk contains about 120 milligrams of calcium per 8-ounce glass. But in the past 15 years, our milk consumption per person has been decreasing, while our cola beverage consumption has increased. Cola beverages contain lots of phosphorus and no calcium. This lowers the calcium-to-phosphorus ratio even further; almost to the proportion that caused secondary hyperparathyroidism in laboratory studies.

What can we do to make sure our calcium-to-phosphorus ratios are correct, and that we get enough calcium? It is possible to treat meat differently to dissolve part of the bone and give us more calcium; marinating the meat would do this trick. Or we can take a calcium supplement. The least expensive way would be to take bone meal or dolomite, which is calcium magnesium carbonate. Supplementation with minerals should be based on the amounts you are already getting in

your foods; 300 to 600 milligrams of calcium should be sufficient for most people. This supplement would also balance
the low calcium content of foods like fish, because we remove
every piece of bone from such foods. I have always warned
against weight-loss plans that urge people to consume only
large amounts of protein and water, because such a diet can
easily cause hyperparathyroidism.

Another way to give our bodies plenty of calcium would be
to drink sufficient quantities of milk, about two to three
glasses per day, preferably skimmed or raw. Recent studies
implicating homogenized milk as a possible cause of heart
disease make raw and skim milk seem much more desirable
as a regular part of the diet.

Dr. Kurt A. Oster, a cardiac specialist at Harvard Medical
School, came to this conclusion after he and some of his
colleagues found the enzyme xanthine oxidase (XO) in the
heart and artery tissue of people who had died of heart attacks. XO is found in milk. When milk is homogenized, the fat
in it is changed into very fine droplets that can move through
the walls of the digestive tract and carry the XO right into the
blood stream, where it attacks the walls of our arteries. The
body, in its attempt to "bandage" the damage, deposits fat
and cholesterol on the weakened tissue. As this process continues, increasing amounts of fat and cholesterol build up,
narrowing the vessels until they can no longer carry enough
blood.

Since heat destroys XO, you can help protect your arteries
by bringing homogenized milk to the boiling point after you
purchase it. We should also encourage the milk industry to
heat milk to higher temperatures during pasteurization, since
normal flash-heating pasteurization temperatures will not kill
the XO.

In raw milk the fat droplets are larger, and the absorption
process is a little different, so XO doesn't make it into the

blood stream. Some supermarkets and health food stores carry raw milk. Skimmed milk has no fat, and therefore no XO.

LACK OF EXERCISE

Exercise plays an extremely important role in the prevention of atherosclerosis. Dr. J. N. Morris and his colleagues at the London School of Hygiene and Tropical Medicine examined the habits of nearly 17,000 middle-aged business executives and office workers and found that those who did vigorous exercises had a much lower rate of heart attacks than those who exercised little or not at all. In a similar study, Dr. Per Bjoerntorp and his associates at the University of Goeteborg in Sweden found that physically well-trained men had an improved carbohydrate metabolism. Further research results published by Dr. Morris indicate that the best possible CHD protection through exercise is achieved when vigorous activity is carried out for at least 30 minutes at a time, rather than more often in shorter periods.

Dr. Herbert DeVries of the University of Southern California studied the exercise habits of older people and found that women and men can improve the fitness of their hearts and blood vessels through systematic physical exercise. He demonstrated that it is wrong for older people to take it easy and avoid difficult exercises. They should stay active as long as possible, allowing common sense to determine a wise level of exertion.

Besides stimulating endocrine functions, the pulsating movement of arteries during exercise increases the circulation of fluids to the cells, and removes the cross-links that make arteries rigid. Naturally, when essential nutrients are not present in the blood, all the exercise in the world won't help. But a program combining exercise and nutrition is a strong weapon against aging.

A AND B PERSONALITY TYPES

Recently there has been a lot of talk about the "Type A" person, who is tense, always on the go, a perfectionist, and a good candidate for an early heart attack. "Type B" people are calmer, more relaxed, and less susceptible to heart attacks. (This theory was first presented in *Type A Behavior and Your Heart*, by Drs. Meyer Friedman and Ray Rosenman.)

In order to find out if such "type casting" is valid, Dr. David C. Jenkins of the Boston University School of Medicine studied 2,750 men who had never had heart attacks. Dr. Jenkins determined, by a questionnaire, the personality group to which each man belonged. After observing the men for four years, he found that Type A men had twice as many heart attacks as Type B.

Type A people are obviously more often under distress, and the importance of distress in contributing to heart attacks is well established.

COFFEE

Our old friend coffee made heart attack news again recently when Dr. Hershel Jick surveyed 12,759 patients and found a correlation between coffee drinking and heart attacks. For heavy coffee drinkers, the risk of heart attack was found to be 120 percent above normal. Since Dr. Jick could not find the same correlation for tea drinkers, he ruled out caffeine as the actual cause. Other studies indicate that coffee is associated with a fast-paced, stress-filled lifestyle, whereas tea is more

147

often part of a relaxed, low-stress approach. It may be for this reason, at least in part, that coffee drinkers are more likely to suffer from heart disease.

SALT AND HIGH BLOOD PRESSURE

An inherited defect that can lead to high blood pressure is the build up of salt in the body. Dr. Lewis K. Dahl of the Brookhaven National Laboratory found that regular table salt can trigger hypertension (high blood pressure) in many people. While white Americans eat about 10 grams of salt per day, black Americans take in twice as much—and have twice as much hypertension. Eskimos eat only 4 grams of salt daily and have almost no hypertension. Dr. Dahl recommends that we limit our salt intake to 5 grams per day, and that people who have a history of high blood pressure in their families limit their salt intake to about 2 grams per day.

Another shocking health report came from Dr. R. Miller, chairman of the Pediatrics Department of Cook County Hospital in Chicago. After evaluating a study of 12,000 suburban high-school students, he found that 16 to 20 out of every 1,000 students had an elevated blood pressure that could be life-threatening by the time they reach middle age. The dividing line was set at a blood pressure of 150/90, which is high for people of this age group; 120/80 plus or minus a few points is generally accepted as a healthy range for adults.

Improving nutrition and lowering salt intake are good measures to start with, and people who take large amounts of vitamin C should use ascorbic acid instead of the sodium ascorbate often found in chewable vitamin C formulations. Let us keep in mind that lowering the blood pressure does not lower the risk of getting diseases of the arteries, but it will certainly decrease the chance of dying from heart disease or stroke.

SMOKING

All other factors being equal, smoking increases your chance of dying from a heart attack by about 600 to 800 percent if you are in the age group 45 to 60. The reason for this can be multifold: One important consideration is that smoking exposes the body to toxic chemicals including oxidants that, when inhaled, will damage our blood vessels first. Also, the carbon monoxide in cigarette smoke reacts with the iron in the blood to reduce its oxygen-carrying capacity. One thing is sure: If we have an already limited blood supply to a vital organ like the heart or brain, the reduced oxygen-carrying capacity due to smoking cigarettes can mean the difference between life and death. Taking large amounts of antioxidants is only a partial solution.

DISHWASHING DETERGENTS

A build up of fat in the liver is strongly associated with heart disease and possibly even cancer. We have also learned that normal functioning of the liver is of the utmost importance for detoxification of the body and for dealing with sugar problems.

Dr. Hans Nieper, head of a large hospital in Hanover, Germany, and a member of health advisory boards in many countries, was one of the first to suggest that dishwashing detergents play a role in the formation of a fatty liver.

Dishwashing detergents contain large polymeric compounds that are not completely removed from the dishes by rinsing with water. The liver can't metabolize these large molecules sufficiently, and their accumulation leads to a buildup of fat.

To protect yourself from this possible danger, use either regular liquid soap (different from detergents and sold in only a few stores) or the organic natural formulations sold in health-food stores. Organic dishwashing fluid is also available in health-food stores.

Chelation Therapy

Often, when people have ruined their health through bad habits, atherosclerosis and arteriosclerosis have advanced to such a degree that good nutrition, even combined with other health factors, is unlikely to help. The doctor then can do very little for the patient. Surgical intervention is enormously expensive, and its results are usually disappointing.

A new treatment uses a compound called ethylenediaminetetraacetic acid (EDTA), which is infused as a solution into the arteries to "flush out" the circulatory system. EDTA binds with mineral ions that are blocking the arteries and dissolves them so they can be removed with the urine. A drawback of this method is that EDTA also binds with almost all other mineral ions, including the desirable ones like copper, manganese, and calcium, removing them as well. If these minerals are immediately replaced, there seems to be no problem. The infusion must be repeated several times, and it can be done in a doctor's office.

Some patients who had arteriosclerosis have shown fantastic improvements after this type of treatment. Many who were almost completely immobilized can walk and move their limbs, and some have played their favorite sports again. Unfortunately drug companies have shown no interest in researching EDTA; perhaps this is because EDTA has been known for a long time and therefore won't yield them any lucrative patents. Doctors who use EDTA are harassed by the FDA and by some medical groups who have no better solutions to offer. This harassment takes the form of negative publicity and, in some cases, threats of license removal. At one point, it led to a court showdown: the judges agreed with the doctors, ruling that when accepted medical practice does not include an adequate solution to a problem, it is not sufficient to do just what everybody else does.

Doctors who practice EDTA and other unorthodox treatments are in the forefront of medical research and they often have important decisions to make when they face the choice of suggesting a new approach to a patient. Doctors in the United States don't have all the freedoms their European counterparts have, and they are always told to follow the generally accepted standard approach.

Many good doctors travel all over the world and learn about new and better methods of treatment. Why should they practice these methods? Because they are great humanitarians? Any deviation from what everybody else practices also leaves them open to malpractice suits, and money-hungry lawyers are willing to make a case out of almost anything. Using a new method of treatment, especially if the standard treatment is highly ineffective, should be left up to the doctor and the patient. Sure, there are also risks in such an approach, but it definitely has its advantages. In Germany, a nation more open to new medical ideas, the death rate from arteriosclerotic heart disease (and other diseases, for example cancer of the colon) is only half of what it is in the United States.

Let's look at another example. If a kidney stone is larger than 9 millimeters, the standard procedure is to operate. Dr. Marion Yandell, a California physician, told me about a patient who had such a kidney stone. The medical consensus was to operate. However, Dr. Yandell was able to remove the stone by applying chelation therapy.

I discussed this method with German doctors during one of my trips to medical meetings. Most authorities agreed that because there is no better treatment for arteriosclerosis, chelation therapy should be used more extensively, and one very conservative doctor even commented that "it sure beats dying." Anyone who wishes further information on chelation therapy in this country can write to: The American Academy of Medical Preventics, 2811 L Street, Sacramento, California 95816.

The Pritikin Approach

During the 1975 Annual Session of the American Congress of Rehabilitation Medicine, and at later meetings of other medical organizations, Nathan Pritikin, director of the Longevity Research Institute at Santa Barbara, California, reported on a tremendously successful treatment for the rehabilitation of patients with severe peripheral vascular disease. The treatment, studied at the Longevity Research Institute in Santa Barbara, California, consisted of a combined diet and exercise program. The main exercise was walking, and the diet consisted of 10 percent protein, 10 percent fat, and 80 percent "complex" carbohydrates (foods as grown). The diet included no refined or simple carbohydrates, such as sugar or honey, and no cholesterol or additional salt. The patients on this program showed tremendous improvements. Their exercise capacity increased and, in many cases, x-rays showed that atherosclerosis had actually been reversed.

This approach eliminates literally all the contributing factors to heart disease I have listed, and the good results are undeniable. However, for several reasons, I do not support this program for long-term use.

152

First, the low protein intake does not reflect latest findings in aging research suggesting that one out of every five calories should come from protein. Other results, from research into depression and the control center in the brain, also indicate such a low protein intake may be undesirable.

Second, though probably beneficial for most patients with certain types of vascular disease, the fat level in this diet is too low for people who get plenty of physical activity.

Third, though this diet would definitely increase vitamin and mineral intake, what would happen if someone on the program returned to his or her normal environment and these quality foods were not available every day? I would be especially concerned about the resulting drop in vitamin consumption. In addition, it is very likely that the calcium level in this diet is too low, or that it induces a calcium-phosphorus imbalance. The diet seems to neglect many important compounds that have been proven helpful for good health.

Your Total Heart Disease Prevention Program

The experts are still arguing over which is the best way to prevent artery and heart disease. Until all the disputes are settled—which could take a long time indeed—the choice is up to us. We can either do everything right, as outlined in this chapter, or we can just do the things that promise the best possible results.

Your personal program might then include:

1). Improving your overall nutrition. Your diet should be high in complex carbohydrates and low in fat, including some, but very little, polyunsaturated fat. (As you increase your extended exercise, you will need more polyunsaturated fat.) Be sure to eat enough protein.

2). Vitamin and mineral supplements. Start with about 500 milligrams of vitamin C and 100 "International Units" (I.U.)

153

of vitamin E, then increase this depending on your needs and other environmental factors. Look for a multivitamin pill with minerals and B-complex vitamins; follow the directions on the bottle. You should adjust your total calcium intake to 1,000 to 1,500 milligrams per day, and your magnesium intake to about 400 to 600 milligrams. But before you begin any vitamin or mineral supplementation program be sure to read Chapter 14 and the Table of Precautions that follows it.

3). An exercise program. Walking at an accelerated pace is good, but jogging is better. Get physical therapy and massages if you can't exercise.

4). Weight reduction, if you're overweight. As a number one priority, you should reduce calories and increase exercise to shed those extra pounds.

5). Learning to deal with distress, or avoiding it if you can't adjust to it.

6). Cutting down on (or cutting out) coffee consumption.

7). Using soap or organic cleansers instead of detergents.

8). No smoking.

9). Using nonfat or raw milk instead of homogenized milk.

10). Having your triglycerides checked by your doctor; if you are overweight, you might wait until you have shed the pounds.

Adjust the variables depending on your environment and individuality. For instance, if your triglycerides are far above 100, increase your exercise, lower your fat intake, and have the blood analysis repeated after three weeks. You'll find that as triglycerides drop, so will the cholesterol level. And while you are fighting heart disease and slowing down your rate of aging, you'll be feeling better as well.

Chapter 12

Preventing Cancer

As one of the cancer researchers put it: "The evidence for a human cancer virus is so strong, I would take any bet that soon we will find and identify it."

After cardiovascular disease, cancer ranks as the second most frequent cause of death in the United States, accounting for about 20 percent of our fatalities in any given year. The incidence of cancer is at an all-time high and shows no signs of decreasing. Strangely enough, experts predicted the current cancer epidemic as long as 30 years ago, but little progress has been made toward preventing it.

Although we have made advances in treating cancer, the survival rate is still not very optimistic. And although the exact cause of cancer has not yet been identified, we do know many of the contributing factors. Once again, I find myself recommending a Multi-Factorial Approach, combining a variety of preventive measures, as the best way of avoiding this life-shortening, age-hastening disease.

The Mechanism of Cancer

The human body consists of communities of cells, many of which are capable of self-renewal by splitting. Cell divisions occur in a series of distinct phases that are the same for normal and neoplastic, or abnormal, cells.

Abnormal growth occurs when one or more cells starts dividing at an unusual rate, and a small tumor forms. This process is called neoplasm. If the tumor is benign, it is usually a local growth, restricted to one area and separated from the neighboring tissue. If it is malignant, or cancerous, it will grow into adjacent tissues. Cancer cells may also break loose and spread to form new tumors somewhere else in the body. This process is called metastasis.

Cancer and Viruses

Although research attempts to pinpoint viruses as the cause of human cancer are not yet conclusive, in animal studies cancer viruses are well established. There are many reasons why a viral cause of human neoplasm could go unrecognized. It could be that viruses cause neoplasm under some conditions but can also infect cells without ill effects. Neoplasm may be caused by viruses that are so common as to be hard to identify. A virus that has induced neoplasm may, when studied by usual methods, have disappeared. Or the techniques for identifying animal viruses may not be applicable to human studies.

Many experts feel that we are very close to having conclusive proof that viruses are the primary cause of cancer. As one researcher put it: "The evidence for a human cancer virus is so strong, I would take any bet that soon we will find and identify it."

I propose that the cancer-causing virus, or the microorganism as proposed by Dr. Virginia Livingston in San Diego, is all around us and that a well functioning immune system keeps it under control. If a cell becomes cancerous, a healthy immune system kills it. But if the immune system malfunctions, or if the amount of carcinogens is too high for it to handle, a tumor forms. Any change toward a more normal system that occurs during the early stages of the cancer would then lead toward its elimination.

The Key: Your Immune System

Once a cell becomes cancerous, a chemical change on its surface alarms our immune system. The warriors in battle against disease are the white blood cells, called lymphocytes, that are made primarily in the bone marrow. Some lymphocytes pass through the thymus gland, where they get a special assignment: They become T-cells, and their function is to attack and kill everything harmful from bacteria to viruses and cancer cells. Other lymphocytes become B-cells which release antibodies against the toxic materials given off by microorganisms or cancer cells. For example, if a bacterial infection takes place, the bacterium itself might not do us any harm, but it may give off toxic wastes. The B-cells will react by making antibodies to deactivate the toxins, and the T-cells kill the bacteria. Likewise, if malignant growth occurs, in a healthy immune system the B-cells' antibodies will deactivate the compounds on the cancer cell surfaces, while the T-cells attack and kill the cancer cells themselves.

The immune system's reactions take time, because the T-cells' function is slower than that of the B-cells. As we age, the T-cell function slows down even more, but there is evidence that it can be stimulated again (the recent discovery of the hormone thymidine looks very promising). This finding is significant, because it has been shown that B- and T-cells must work together for an effective system.

SUPPORTING STUDIES

Dr. W. H. Adler reported to the 1973 Symposium on Theoretical Aspects of Aging, in Miami, that when cancer cells were transplanted into mice, they continued to grow if only the B-cells were attacking them. If the T-cells were intact, and provoked to action, the cancer was killed.

At Roosevelt University in Chicago, I achieved good life extensions on animals with the use of RN-13 nucleic acid injections, which are being used in Germany on humans. A few months ago, it was demonstrated that nucleic acid injections can stimulate the formation of interferon, a key factor in speeding the responses of our immune system to cancer. If the immune system is slow to respond, cancer cells keep dividing unhindered and a tumor may grow to such a size that immune therapy is ineffective, and surgery is necessary.

A CANCER CASE HISTORY

About three years ago, a friend of mine called me from Atlanta and wanted to know if I had any suggestions about further treatment of his mother, who had just had a radical mastectomy. I asked him to send me a copy of her medical history and I made a few phone calls to friends who were also doing work in cancer-related fields. It looked very bad; the cancer had spread to over 90 percent of the lymph tissue and the patient was given a 15 percent chance of surviving six months. My friend still wanted to go ahead and try anything he could.

At first we improved the woman's diet, put her on megavitamins and minerals, and suggested digestive enzymes. Then we flew her to San Diego for an appointment with Dr. Virginia Livingston, who has spent her life studying cancer and who has, with other doctors, developed a vaccine to stimulate the immunity system to fight cancer. From Dr. Livingston, the patient first received a BCG (Bacillus Calmette Guerin) vaccination, and blood and urine samples were taken to prepare another kind of immunity stimulant vaccine which Dr. Livingston had been working with for years. The patient also received an antibiotic and gammaglobulin shots.

The next step was to evaluate all her habits and look for possible causes of cancer. Quality foods like brewer's yeast, liver, and wheat germ oil were incorporated in her diet, which emphasized a low fat and sugar intake. Then we checked environmental factors. Alcohol consumption was slightly decreased, a minor possible distress situation was eliminated, exercise (walking) was increased, and the air she inhaled (polluted with cigarette smoke) was improved. Another German vaccine was added to the list, and after a few weeks of recuperation she went back to Turkey, where she was living at the time.

The regimen outlined above was continued with only minor variations. Six months, and then one year later, examinations showed that things looked fine. Two years later she was back in the United States to visit her son in Atlanta. No signs of cancer. Three years after the operation, when she was given a 15 percent chance to survive six months, she was back in the United States again and her health was good.

The principle behind this successful case history was to do literally everything to support her immune system, and to eliminate all possible causes of cancer.

Prevention of Cancer

To prevent cancer in healthy persons, or to hamper its recurrence after surgery or other treatments, we can combine three major approaches that will simultaneously help to delay aging:

1. Supporting the body's defenses as well as possible with superb nutrition and health habits.

2. Reactivation of immune responses with vaccines from time to time.

3. Elimination of as many cancer-causing agents as possible.

All of these factors are so important that it's difficult to say which should be given the highest priority. Super nutrition and good health habits have already been explained in Part II of this book.

Some of the vaccines that can stimulate our immune system are BCG, the Kryptocides vaccines developed by Dr. Virginia Livingston in San Diego and Dr. Chisato Maruyama in Japan, a vaccine against breast cancer developed by Dr. James Charney in Camden, New Jersey, and a stomach cancer vaccine developed by Drs. Eugene Edynak, Noboru Oishi, and Benjamin Gordon in Hawaii. Other vaccines against lung cancer and cancer of the lymphatic system are being worked on in Canada and in Germany.

BCG, originally used against tuberculosis, had earlier been found to stimulate immune responses in humans and animals. When the importance of the immune system became clear in the treatment of cancer, BCG was investigated at various levels of cancer research. When vaccinated with BCG, animals show a much higher resistance to cancer cells.

BCG is used by an increasing number of doctors here in the United States. For referral to doctors in various parts of the United States who are using BCG, the Research Foundation,

70 W. Hubbard Street, Chicago, Illinois 60610 will supply information.

Cell injections are also used to stimulate immune responses. One of these preparations was developed by Cybila Laboratorien in Heidelberg, Germany, and is sold in Germany under the name of Resistocell.

Three vitamins (A, C, and E), and a mineral (selenium, in trace amounts) have been linked with increased immune functions, as discussed in Chapter 13. Dr. Karl Ransberger in Munich has achieved excellent results with cancer patients who were given 1.5 to 3 million units of vitamin A per day in a special emulsion. Medical supervision of this treatment is vital, as vitamin A can be toxic in large doses.

Many of the contributing factors to cancer—which, of course, are also some of the major causes of aging—seem to be linked with certain chemical processes in the body. Three types of compounds are important in understanding these "oxidation" reactions:

1). Some compounds can be oxidized in our body to form carcinogens. The nitrogen-containing compounds ranging from antibiotics to pesticides, and even some of the essential nutrients like amino acids, would fall in this category.

2). Other compounds can oxidize the compounds listed above to form carcinogens, for example: nitrites, nitrates, ozone, and oxidants in cigarette smoke and air pollution.

3). Then we have antioxidants, which can prevent oxidation reactions. Among these are vitamins C and E, the mineral selenium, and synthetic antioxidants like the food additives BHT and BHA. Certainly I would rather see the use of natural antioxidants, but in longevity studies, and in some cancer studies on humans and animals, these synthetic antioxidants have shown some very positive effects.

161

THE MAJOR CONTRIBUTING FACTORS

In discussing the major cancer-causing factors, one would have to include among the risks smoking, faulty nutrition, lack of vitamins and minerals, lack of exercise, and food additives like nitrates and nitrites.

When a connection between animal fats and heart attacks was found a few years ago, many people started to replace these fats with plant oils. Polyunsaturates are important, but to shift the intake of fats too heavily toward them and away from animal fat can actually increase the cancer risk, according to several medical reports.

A high fat intake is often the cause for being overweight and for having high triglyceride levels. High triglyceride levels cause blood cells to clump together, and this reduces the blood's oxygen-carrying ability. Since good oxygen transport is an essential requirement for cancer prevention, being overweight and having high triglycerides are also established as cancer risk factors.

Vitamin B 15, whose major function is to increase the oxygen availability in the blood, thus gains increased importance when the oxygen-carrying capacity of the blood is reduced for other reasons. Russian researchers have also demonstrated that B 15 plays an important role in preventing premature aging.

Dr. Hans Selye and other researchers have demonstrated that distress can hamper immune responses, making it another possible risk factor. This topic is covered in Chapter 8.

Environmental pollutants also contribute to the formation of cancer, and here again the synergistic factor arises. Professor Irving Selikoff, Director of the Environmental Sciences Laboratory at the Mt. Sinai School of Medicine in New York, has found that a combination of cigarette smoke and air pollution can be highly dangerous, and that asbestos workers who smoke have an 800 percent increased cancer risk.

At Baylor Medical College, Drs. Wan-Bang Lo and Homer S. Black found that when we are exposed to the sun for long periods, ultraviolet light causes the cholesterol in skin cells to be converted into cholesterol oxide, a known carcinogen. Vitamins C and E can prevent this reaction and thus might be important in the prevention of skin cancer and other types of cancer.

Many aerosol sprays contain chlorinated hydrocarbons as propellants; the connection between these compounds and cancer is quite strong. Avoid using aerosols whenever possible. Chlorinated hydrocarbons are also used as dry-cleaning fluids and as the raw materials for many plastic bottles. In July 1977, a National Cancer Institute spokesman disclosed that this solvent caused liver cancer in about half of the 200 mice tested. Therefore, air your dry-cleaned clothes well before you wear them.

Aromatic hydrocarbons, found in high percentages in the oily mess one often steps in when walking along a beach, must either be oxidized within the body or acted upon by the enzyme AHH (Aryl Hydrocarbon Hydroxylase) before they become true carcinogens. Since AHH is found in the human body, this particular mechanism for cancer formation is well established. (And, since AHH levels vary from person to person, those with high levels of the enzyme can help protect themselves from cancer by being especially careful to avoid aromatic hydrocarbons.) Beach tars, which result from oil spills at sea, are also high in aromatic compounds that contribute to skin cancer formation. The oil industry would be well advised to spend more of its millions cleaning up these messes than it does on TV commercials expressing concern for the environment. Aromatic hydrocarbons are also in crude oil. It is therefore amazing to see that industry dares to suggest the construction of an oil terminal in Long Beach,

163

California, which would add the equivalent pollution of 2.7 million automobiles to the already dangerous air of this area.

Several types of radiation, including medical x-rays, have been associated with cancer formation, probably because they cause the formation of free radicals. (These abnormal molecules are involved in cancer formation.) Therefore, it is wise to avoid unnecessary x-rays. Mention your concern to your doctor.

In Chapter 3 we saw the importance of super nutrition in the overall anti-aging program, and diet is crucial in the prevention of cancer. Recent findings showed that fiber in our food is the major factor in avoiding colon-rectal cancer. Professor Denis Burkitt, an English surgeon and Nobel Prize recipient, demonstrated that increasing the fiber content of the diet accelerates the movement of foods through the digestive tract, preventing the build up of carcinogens there.

Saccharin has been implicated many times as a contributing factor to cancer formation; to clarify this point many studies are still being done. A combined study of the National Cancer Institute of Canada and researchers at several Canadian universities concluded that male users of artificial sweeteners, including saccharin and cyclamate, had a 60 percent greater chance of getting bladder cancer than men who didn't use them.

Avoid the use of these sweeteners! As demonstrated in the study I discussed in Chapter 4, not even diabetics need these sweeteners. They can deal with their problem in other ways.

Food additives are also under investigation as a probable cancer factor. At the University of Nebraska Medical Center in Omaha, scientists studied the reactions between the common additives nitrates and nitrites and "amino group" chemicals found in many foods and natural compounds in our body. Though essential as ingredients for "amino acids," "amino group" chemicals can also react with nitrites and nitrates to form nitrosamine compounds, known carcinogens. The University of Nebraska at Omaha researchers found that vitamin C blocks the formation of these nitrosamines, again underscoring the importance of vitamin C in cancer prevention. But why should we take this risk in the first place? There is no need for cancer-causing chemicals in our foods. All they do is help big food producers increase their profits at the expense of your health.

HOW MUCH IS TOO MUCH?

Each time someone discovers a new carcinogen that we take into our bodies in small quantities, through food or drinking water, some expert will step forward and declare that "in such negligible amounts" the chemical does not represent a cancer hazard. From where do these experts get the wisdom to make statements unsupported by scientific facts?

In one experiment, we subjected mice to a mixture of several such carcinogens in "safe" quantities. The chemicals used were nitrites, nitrates, DES, saccharin, and Chicago tap water. A control group received none of the above; its drinking fluid consisted of spring water purchased at a local supermarket. Results: the treated animals had an average lifespan 20 percent shorter than the controls, mainly due to an increase in cancer.

The trouble with "safe" quantities of carcinogens is that, in combination with "safe" quantities of other carcinogens, they are highly dangerous. This synergistic mutual reinforcement by the various cancer factors has been demonstrated many times in scientific studies, yet it is very often overlooked.

Some Facts About Breast Cancer

In the light of the many contributing factors, it is astonishing to see that so little is done about preventing this disease.

An increase in cancer overall, and in ovarian and breast cancer specifically, was associated by researchers in England, the United States, Germany, and Russia with a high animal-fat intake. This is also a well-established contributing factor to heart disease, diabetes, and other serious health problems. Any health-promoting or cancer-preventing program should start by lowering triglycerides, removing some of the excess fat from the diet, and achieving a normal weight.

A few years ago some German doctors found that when female hormones were metabolized at a normal speed, there was little breast cancer. But when the speed of hormone metabolism wasn't normal, a higher incidence of breast cancer was observed. Furthermore, when they tried to find out what substances helped to normalize this metabolism rate, they discovered the B-vitamins were responsible. For this reason, women should make sure they receive enough B-vitamins in their diets. Some birth control pill manufacturers already include B-vitamins in their formulations.

Exercise helps control triglycerides and it also stimulates metabolism of hormones. Nothing new! So this is also part of the plan to prevent breast cancer.

The role of antioxidants in the reduction of cancer rates is well established, and the same finding is true for breast cancer. In addition, vitamin A and the mineral selenium are important in combating breast cancer. A statistically recognized decrease in breast cancer has been recorded in areas where the selenium content of the soil, and therefore also of the food, is higher. Selenium is also used in Germany in the treatment of cancer.

Environmental factors like air pollution and chemicals in

the drinking water should naturally be avoided to prevent breast cancer, and this brings us back to the importance of good health habits and nutrition in eliminating many cancer-causing factors from our lives.

IF BREAST CANCER SHOULD HAPPEN TO YOU

Since a radical mastectomy is such a crude procedure and one which greatly affects the entire life and psychological well-being of a woman, many surgeons consider the local removal of a tumor rather than a radical removal of the whole breast. This, however, decreases survival rates. In order to find the lowest risk approach, I have discussed this with many doctors in the field of cancer and preventive medicine. We were able to reach reasonable agreement for the following approach which will vary from person to person, depending on her history, size of tumor, and other factors:

1. Super nutrition with large amounts of vitamins C, E, and A, and digestive enzymes, including trace amounts of selenium, and no smoking, at least for a few days before BCG vaccination. When administered to an undernourished body, BCG might cause a breakdown of the entire system. It's like revving up an engine that doesn't have any oils or lubricants; you'll burn it up for sure.

2. Possibly, application of another vaccine like the breast cancer vaccines or the Livingston vaccine before surgery is performed. These vaccines will activate immune responses so cancer cells that might break loose during surgery are destroyed.

3. If possible, surgical removal of only the tumor itself. This should be followed by gamma globulin shots, metavitamins, super nutrition, excellent health habits, chemotherapy, antibiotics, and other measures.

167

This special section on breast cancer has been included because so many surgeons rarely consider the feelings of a woman when a radical mastectomy is recommended; because I myself feel very strongly about this new approach; because it has very little chance of hurting anyone; and because similar combined approaches have shown success against other types of cancer.

LAETRILE

When laetrile, the controversial cancer drug, becomes available, I will include it in the program to prevent recurrence of any type of cancer. Several good studies demonstrate beneficial effects of this drug, but I would rather look at it as a supporting drug that should be included in a total approach. In Germany, researchers have gone much further with this type of drug and have tested new derivatives which could be even better.

Laetrile is very inexpensive and, if applied in the right amounts, has no negative side effects. Whether to use it should be up to the doctor and patient.

That a multi-factorial approach is also necessary for treatments involving laetrile was demonstrated by Dr. Harold Manner at Loyola University in Chicago. In one of his studies, mice were treated successfully against breast cancer with a combination of laetrile, vitamins, and enzymes.

If the FDA has evidence that it is of doubtful merit, doctors should be so informed and further tests should be performed under conditions which would satisfy the supporters and the opponents. But until a true cure for cancer becomes available, laetrile should be included in our methods of treatment.

The Case of Richard M.

In closing this chapter, let me cite the case history of a patient with a terminal cancer who recovered so fast that the medical profession called it "one of those miraculous recoveries without scientific explanation." But, as we'll see, there is an explanation.

Richard M. was a baker's helper in Germany. When he went for a medical checkup one day, the doctor called his employer and told him that Richard had an advanced lung cancer and that it was a miracle he had lived so long. Could the employer give him a special vacation so the man could live out his last few weeks doing something he always wanted to enjoy?

Richard got a bonus "for being such a good employee and for helping to make the business a success" and took off for the Bavarian Alps, not knowing he had only a few weeks to live. He was given the address of a hospital where he was to check in from time to time.

At the bakery, his co-workers were waiting for the bad news to come that Richard had died, but instead he kept writing excited letters about living in the mountains and how well he was feeling. He said he had met a doctor who gave him hell for smoking, and so he quit. He enjoyed the clean air and the good food available in the mountains, and in order to cut down on costs he picked berries and mushrooms and learned about herbs and natural foods.

"When do you want me to come back?" he kept asking in his letters. His employer found all kinds of excuses to let him have "one more" week in his new paradise, which had only been a dream when Richard used to get up at 3 A.M. to start his shift in the bakery.

Eventually hospital testing showed that Richard's cancer had been localized and was actually shrinking. It is now 18 years later. Richard is still working in the bakery, and saving

169

money so he can spend some time in the mountains each year.

A miracle? Definitely not. There is a logical explanation for Richard's recovery. He quit smoking, thus eliminating a major cancer hazard. He reduced his distress, and his body was better able to combat the disease. Nutrition and clean air and water also helped to support his immune responses. The case of Richard M. fits right into the Multi-Factorial Approach to fighting cancer.

The Future

The chances for finding a true cure for cancer are very good, because promising results are already being achieved in many different avenues of research. In one area, scientists have already found some ways to change cancer cells back into normal cells. In other experiments, the growth of cancer cells was dramatically affected by subjecting the host of cancer cells to mixtures of different gases under different pressures.

But even when we find a cancer cure, preventive medicine will still be better than suffering through the disease and a cure which is likely to be unpleasant. A body kept healthy through good habits is not only more resistant to cancer; it is also more resistant to other diseases and to the aging process itself. Again the key is prevention—with a Multi-Factorial Approach.

Chapter 13

Preventing Senility and Other Mental Disorders

"Of all the problems associated with advanced age, surely senile dementia is the most tragic; the effects are devastatingly depersonalizing and ultimately dehumanizing."

Robert T. Terry, M.D.
Henryk M. Wisniewski, M.D., Ph.D.
140th Meeting, American Association
for the Advancement of Science,
February, 1974

In the previous two chapters, we discussed prevention of circulatory diseases and cancer. To round out the anti-aging program, this chapter will discuss the changes in the brain associated with aging, and what we can do to fight them.

Aging and the Brain

The central nervous system includes the brain and the spinal cord, and it is subdivided into gray and white matter. When we talk about the brain, we actually mean that part of

171

the nervous system contained in the skull. Here we have billions of nerve cells with a total weight of approximately 1,380 grams for a man and 1,250 grams for a woman. ("Which proves," as a female friend of mine puts it, "intelligence does not depend on the size of the brain.")

As we age, we lose thousands of brain cells every day. In terms of the total number of brain cells available, this loss is not so dramatic, because we use only a small part of the brain. However, according to my Combination Theory on Aging, the loss of cells is not merely a symptom of aging; it *is* aging. If we can prevent a loss of cells, we will have delayed the aging process as well.

More than just the overall cell loss in the brain is important, because other major control organs are also located in the skull. Two of them are the thalamus and the hypothalamus. The thalamus is a relay center for several kinds of sensory impulses, including temperature variations and pain. The hypothalamus regulates temperature and metabolism; it also controls secretions of the anterior pituitary gland and thus rules normal sexual functions. These organs are of special importance because they appear to be involved in the control center in the brain.

Until just a short time ago, the pituitary was considered the major control organ, but the discovery of the neuroendocrines showed that the hypothalamus controls the pituitary. Some of the control mechanisms in the hypothalamus suggest that it might very well be possible to make the brain function at levels comparable to its younger days merely by affecting the balance of chemicals in it.

Understanding Senility

A few of the earlier signs of senility, or senile dementia, are slowed thinking processes, slight speech disturbances, and impaired judgment. Until recently it was believed that senility was caused mainly by diseases of the arteries, which limited the supply of oxygen and nutrients to the brain, but medical opinions on this subject are rapidly changing. Studies have demonstrated a decreased blood flow to the brain of senile people, but only 15 to 20 percent of senility is actually caused by diseases of the arteries. An additional 7 percent is caused by syphilis, brain trauma, and tumors. But what is the cause of the remaining approximate 70 percent?

We now have indications that shrinkage of the brain tissue is the answer. Dr. Robert Terry of the Albert Einstein College of Medicine recently reported that in most cases of senility the brain has lost "at least 15 percent and often up to about 30 percent" of its normal weight. And if we look at the neurons (the nerve cells) alone, we find that up to the age of about 85, up to 50 percent are lost. Brain cells don't divide, and we have only a limited number of them available. Lost cells are not replaced. But we can, to a significant extent, prevent an abnormal loss of brain cells.

Keeping Brain Cells in the Best of Health

The brain is made up of very sophisticated cells that, on the average, have a very low storage capacity of nutrients, vitamins, and minerals. Therefore, any shortage of these essential compounds will hamper brain operations. To assure the best possible brain functioning, we must bathe these cells at all times in body fluids that contain the right amounts of all the required nutrients; an excess of one will not make up for the lack of another.

Is there proof that improved nutrition is related to an improved mental health profile? This question can be answered with a definite "yes." Animal experiments have indicated this relationship for some time, and now Dr. E. Cheraskin, of the

University of Alabama, has shown that the same is true of humans.

Dr. Cheraskin reported to the International Academy of Preventive Medicine in 1975 the results of a study indicating that nutrition, in particular vitamins and minerals, can strongly reduce psychological problems. "The subjects with the better psychological scores show higher intake of practically all nutrients, with one exception, namely refined carbohydrates." Health magazines like *Prevention, Let's Live,* and *Bestways* have taken this stand for years, while the American Medical Association and the Food and Drug Administration have labeled it as quackery. Now many doctors are coming around to good nutrition as the basis for mental as well as physical health.

Additional support for the belief that a nutritional deficiency, especially a deficiency of vitamins, can cause mental illness comes from England. There scientists have found that schizophrenics and manic depressives tend to be born during winter months, when vitamin deficiencies are more likely to occur. The importance of making *all* nutrients available to *all* brain cells at *all* times simply cannot be overemphasized, especially for children.

Abnormal Fibers in the Brain

Two scientists at the Albert Einstein College of Medicine recently uncovered what might be another clue toward discovering a cause of senility. Drs. Robert Terry and Henryk M. Wisniewski focused their attention on "senile plaques," high molecular weight fibers probably left over from dead cells in the brain. The two researchers found that people with senile dementia had a surprisingly high concentration of these plaques, and that in such cases, the plaques consisted of abnormal "twisted tubules" of protein. Terry and Wisniewski suggested that these strange tubules might be formed by one of two mechanisms: a virus, in which case safe antiviral agents such as vitamin C might be able to block tubule formation; or abnormal oxidation reactions, which could be prevented with anti-oxidants such as vitamins C and E. Future research into these fibers may give modern medicine another tool for slowing down aging.

Oxygen and the Brain

One nutrient whose absence in the brain, even for only a few minutes, will cause death, is the simple gas oxygen. For years, doctors have had patients breathe pure oxygen, sometimes in a pressure chamber ("hyperbaric oxygen"), as treatment for a variety of diseases.

Anybody who has taken a scuba diving course has heard about "the bends." When a diver breathing air rather than straight oxygen stays at depths below 30 feet for an extended period, he must take his time and make "decompression stops" on his way back to the surface. If the diver does not have enough air to make these stops and is forced to ascend faster, that's when the trouble starts. Because of the higher pressure under water, some of the nitrogen in the air he inhaled dissolves in his fatty tissue. The stops for decompression let this nitrogen escape from fatty tissue slowly. If the diver ascends too fast, the nitrogen starts to form bubbles. Besides causing pain, the bubbles can destroy important cells and tissues in the body. This is called "the bends." To push the nitrogen bubbles back into the fatty tissue, and then release them very slowly, a diver with the bends is placed in a decompression chamber filled with air.

HYPERBARIC OXYGEN (HBO) TREATMENTS

The same approach, using pure oxygen in a pressure chamber, has been found beneficial for treating burns, gangrene, and even osteomyelitis, a painful infection of the bone marrow. People being treated for such diseases normally spend about 2 hours in a pressure chamber where they inhale pure oxygen at about twice normal atmospheric pressure. The side effects observed during this kind of treatment recently caught the attention of the popular press and of researchers working in gerontology.

An old man who was impotent reported that his sexual capability had returned after undergoing oxygen therapy. A bald soldier found his hair growing back. Others noticed tremendous improvements in alertness and I.Q. levels. When these findings became known, a number of doctors picked up the treatment for their older patients. Oxygen therapy is now being used to treat conditions from senility to circulatory problems.

THE SCIENTIFIC BASIS FOR OXYGEN THERAPY

There is an excellent scientific basis for oxygen treatment. Oxygen is one of the most important essential compounds for the normal functioning of our cells, particularly those of the heart and brain. When the basic ingredients of food are burned in the cells to give energy, the presence of oxygen is a must. Without it energy production in our body would soon cease.

What makes oxygen so advantageous for the aging person?

When we age, diseases of the arteries may seriously limit the oxygen supply to the various tissues. Cells may still live if the oxygen supply is not completely cut off, but their level of functioning may be very low. Getting more oxygen into the blood will allow those cells to function normally again, and a revitalization effect is observed.

More important, oxygen-burning reactions can cleanse old cells of leftovers or other buildups that restrict the oxygen supply. We are not really sure how this works, but it is known that entire enzyme systems depend on the presence of oxygen and that these enzyme systems don't function as well when we get older. Thus oxygen therapy probably clears up some of the blockage that causes a limited oxygen supply. A general improvement of oxygen-requiring metabolic reactions is possible: Anybody who knows metabolic charts will confirm that the possibilities are numerous.

In 1970, HBO was used with some success to treat senility, and later investigations showed it may be even more effective as a preventive measure. Senility can be caused by a restricted blood flow to the brain, which can be counteracted by doses of oxygen. Dr. Eleanor Jacobs, exploring the question of whether HBO could improve memory, at first found remarkable improvements in her subjects. A few years later more patients were examined and more factors were analyzed, leading doctors to conclude that HBO definitely improves memory. However, the duration of the improvement was uncertain.

A FEW WORDS OF CAUTION

The beneficial effect of HBO appears to be generally established. Now we have to consider possible harmful long-term effects. Any time we increase the oxygen content of the blood, the entire body will receive more oxygen. Tissues whose oxygen supply is not impaired and which are functioning normally could actually be harmed by an excess of oxygen.

In our laboratory we subjected animals to pure oxygen for about 30 minutes per day. The animals perked up at first and looked better than the controls, but then they started to die off just a little faster—as if they had burned the candle at both ends.

This experiment indicates that we should be very careful in the application of oxygen therapy. Some appears good, an excess may have drawbacks. Could it be that in our animal experiment much more oxygen than essential nutrients was transported into the cells, and therefore the animals "burned up"? These animals did not get all the vitamin and mineral supplements; they just received a standard diet. Would they have lived longer if they had received a higher quality nutrition in combination with megavitamins? More research will have to clarify this point.

In view of oxygen's importance for the best possible functioning of the brain cells and the heart, the best oxygen therapy is to reduce fat intake, breathe clean air, and quit smoking.

Part IV

Three Giant Steps Toward Dealing with the True Causes of Aging

Scientists are well on their way toward understanding the causing of aging, and discovering how we can slow that process down. At times it seems only one thing stands in the way—money. Much of the money for most health research comes from industry, as grants. But why should the big food processors, the tobacco industry, and the synthetic drug industry commit suicide by financing research in gerontology? So far, longevity studies only indicate that we would have to shut down large parts of these industries.

Chapter 14

A New Concept of Vitamin Requirements—Plus an Added Ingredient

"In over 300 consecutive obstetrical cases, we found that the simple stress of pregnancy increased the ascorbic acid demand up to 15 grams daily. ... Compare this to the 100 milligrams now recommended in pregnancy by the National Academy of Science and National Research Council and the disparity is shocking. Fred Stare's 40 milligrams per day is catastrophic. This must be changed."

Fred R. Klenner, M.D.
Journal of the International Academy of Preventive Medicine,
Spring, 1974 (Vol. I, no. 1), p. 58.

Most people tend to think of vitamins in terms of the Minimum Daily Requirements (MDRs), and Recommended Daily

Allowances (RDAs). When the MDRs were found insufficient for many people, a slight increase in the amounts changed them into the new RDAs. This is the usual way that doctors and laymen alike judge their vitamin intake.

But current developments in the field of nutrition have shown that vitamins have the potential of being much more important, and that our bodies require greater quantities of them, than we have previously realized. Furthermore, in order to work properly, many vitamins require the presence of certain minerals, often referred to as trace elements, in sufficient amounts.

Physicians and scientists have recently been exposed to some astounding cases of megavitamin therapy; cases in which serious diseases, some considered incurable, have been treated successfully with large quantities of vitamins. Such cases also have taught us a great deal about the role of vitamins in so-called healthy people.

Saved By Vitamin C

On September 10, 1973, a 21-year old male student was admitted to the health department at a major university in southern Illinois. He was unconscious, and his life signs were very low. The doctor arranged to have the young man transferred to the Carl Foundation Hospital in Urbana and notified the patient's parents. At the hospital the doctors tried to diagnose the young man's condition. Kidney diseases were ruled out with kidney function tests, meningitis was ruled out by a sugar test on the spinal fluid, a brain tumor was ruled out by a brain scan, and a heart problem was ruled out with an angiogram. This left only viral encephalitis, an inflammation of the brain, as the cause of the illness. A panel of three doctors informed the parents that their son had approximately 24 hours to live.

At this point the father, a biochemist, asked the neurologist in charge to administer massive amounts of vitamin C to the patient, and the doctor agreed. He administered 50 grams (50,000 milligrams) intravenously the first day and 80 grams per day subsequently. Within a few hours the young man's life signs became normal and his unconscious state changed into a restful sleep. In another 8 hours he woke up. After 4 days of treatment the young man was well enough to be taken out of intensive care, but was held there for a fifth day as a precaution. In 8 days he was released from the hospital. At this point tests showed conclusively that the young man had had viral encephalitis.

Since then, the young man has returned to the hospital for frequent examinations. He has shown no evidence of brain damage or muscle impairment, two common afflictions of people who have recovered from viral encephalitis. Another frequent aftereffect of this disease is a long period of suffering from severe headaches, probably caused by broken blood vessels in the brain. This young man had headaches for only a few days. Fortunately for him, his father was familiar with the work of Dr. Fred Klenner of North Carolina, who has had great success in treating diseases with large doses of vitamin C.

Healing With Vitamins

Irwin Stone, biochemist and author of the magnificent book *The Healing Factor, Vitamin C Against Disease,* told me that he has treated canine distemper with vitamin C and achieved a high ratio of recoveries. Distemper, one of the most serious diseases of domestic dogs, is an airborne, highly infectious virus disease that attacks the nervous system, much like viral encephalitis in humans. Before megascorbic therapy (treatment with large quantities of vitamin C, or ascorbic acid), distemper caused a high percentage of fatalities, and animals that recovered from it usually suffered brain damage. Irwin Stone, a noted biochemist, has reduced the mortality rate of canine distemper from 85 percent to about 20 percent by intravenous use of 1 to 2 grams of sodium ascorbate per pound body weight per day.

Cases like this are not unusual in people any more. Treating virus diseases, Dr. Fred Klenner has achieved excellent results with large doses of vitamin C. A man who had chicken pox was cured by taking 30 grams of vitamin C by mouth each day for four days.

The role of vitamin C in preventing atherosclerosis and cancer has been discussed in Chapters 11 and 12. In addition, a statistical study by a British doctor showed that low vitamin C levels in foods were linked to higher mortality rates.

And the evidence for vitamin therapy continues to mount:

In 1973, Drs. Keith Reisinger, Kenneth Rogers, John Coulehan, and Daniel Bradley reported proof that Professor Linus Pauling was correct in his claim that vitamin C can prevent colds. These four doctors studied 641 children at a Navajo boarding school and found that those given 1 to 2 grams of vitamin C per day had about 34 percent fewer days of illness due to colds. Their overall susceptibility to other illnesses also dropped.

In a 1974 article in the Journal of the International Academy of Preventive Medicine, Dr. Fred Klenner explained why vitamin C can reverse chemical shock and completely relieve the symptoms of urethritis.

Vitamin C is also used as one of the compounds in our longevity studies and, besides life extensions, we found a reduction in cancer in the test animals that received large quantities of this vitamin.

At the 1973 Symposium on Preventive Medicine, Dr. Wilfrid Shute presented evidence that scars are smoother and more elastic if they are treated with vitamin E during the healing process.

In 1973, an article in *Chemical and Engineering News* showed that vitamin C and E act synergistically; they enhance each other's function.

In the light of all this information, one wonders how much longer researchers will be asked to demonstrate the positive effects of vitamin C before the reluctant American Medical Association will accept it. During a recent televised panel discussion, Professor Roger Williams, Professor Linus Pauling, and Dr. Wilfrid Shute agreed that about 400 milligrams of vitamin E and 1500 milligrams of vitamin C per day could be very beneficial for the majority of people. But our conservative medical authorities continue to rely on the recommended daily allowances of 30 milligrams a day for vitamin E and 60 milligrams a day for vitamin C as a guideline, thus standing in the way of the many people who could benefit from megavitamin therapy.

Some News About Vitamin A

Most vitamins are water-soluble, which means that if too much of them builds up in our body, the excess will be eliminated quickly in the urine. Vitamin A is different: It is fat soluble, and an excess cannot be disposed of so easily. In large quantities, vitamin A can be toxic. Vitamin A poisoning has been associated with blurred vision, hair loss, itching, skin disorders, and other symptoms.

But how much vitamin A is too much?

The present recommended daily allowance is 5000 international units (IUs). I take a daily supplement of 30,000 units. Dr. Klenner has used 150,000 to 200,000 IUs a day (about 30 to 40 times the RDA) for many years in treating a patient with ichthyosis, a skin disease. Dr. Karl Ramsberger in Germany uses 1,500,000 to 3,000,000 units per day for at least two months in the treatment of cancer.

Professor Roslyn Alfin-Slater, a quite cautious authority on vitamins, has told medical students at UCLA that a person can consume twice the RDA of fat-soluble vitamins and five times the RDA of water-soluble vitamins without danger. Therefore, most normal people could safely take a daily vitamin A supplement of 10,000 units. If you take larger quantities (and I would not advise anybody to go over 30,000 to 50,000 units per day), going one day every week or so without vitamin A supplementation could help your body throw off any excess.

There are some indications that larger amounts of other vitamins—C and E—raise the vitamin A tolerance. But until more information is available, let's stay a little on the conservative side.

NEW VITAMIN A FINDINGS

Recent studies show that vitamin A is more useful than we had ever imagined. For example, in a 1974 article, Thomas H. Maugh summarized several ground-breaking discoveries about vitamin A, all of which have obvious potential for the prevention and treatment of disease. Among the findings he reported were that carcinogens (cancer-causing substances) bind stronger to tissues of vitamin A-deficient animals than to those of healthy animals; that colon tumors were more frequent in animals lacking in vitamin A; and that even in animals receiving normal amounts of vitamin A, extra dosages can be highly protective against cancer.

All the recent studies of our vitamin needs point to one conclusion: the statement often made by conservative "nutrition experts" that "if you eat a balanced diet, you will get all the vitamins you need," is *not* correct.

What practical conclusions can we draw from these research findings? Where is the borderline between maximum performance supplementation and an increased risk to our health?

Again, let us start with our animal model.

Vitamins and Longevity: a Study

One of our longevity studies measured the effect of vitamin and mineral supplementation on the average lifespan of test animals. Since exercise is an essential requirement and might affect vitamin requirements, it was also a factor in the study. The test animals received wheat germ, brewer's yeast, and large amounts of vitamin and mineral supplements. Vitamin C was added to the drinking water in increasing amounts, reaching a peak equivalent to 4,000 milligrams per day in a human. Vitamin A was equivalent to 20,000 to 30,000 IUs per day. Another supplement the test animals received contained vitamins B_1, B_2, B_3, B_6, and B_{12}, along with other members of the B-vitamin group, in amounts about 30 times higher than in the standard diet. The animals were fed dolomite (calcium and magnesium) equivalent to a human daily intake of about 600 milligrams of calcium and 380 milligrams of magnesium. The average vitamin E intake was equivalent to about 100 to 200 IUs a day for a human. All these supplements were given in addition to what is considered a normal and complete diet for these animals.

Results: Average life extensions ranged from 45 percent to 65 percent. No negative side effects were observed.

We used such high levels of supplements to discover whether a true excess of vitamins would do any harm. It apparently didn't. Since we have shown in animal tests that a thirty-fold excess of vitamins does no harm, a ten-fold increase in the water soluble vitamins and a two- to three-fold increase in the fat-soluble vitamins should pose very little risk for humans.

Human Vitamin Needs

We don't have to rely on animal experiments alone; proof is already available that human vitamin needs are far above what the FDA tells us. During the 1975 September meeting of the International Academy of Preventive Medicine, Professor E. Cheraskin reported some truly startling results. Working with doctors and their wives throughout the state of Alabama, Dr. Cheraskin tried to discover the relation between vitamin intake and overall health. He found that the healthiest subjects consumed an average of 410 milligrams per day of vitamin C, over nine times the RDA; 32,000 units of vitamin A, or about six times the recommended allowance; and about 115 milligrams of niacin (vitamin B$_3$), or five to six times the RDA.

Even though they don't deal with all the vitamins, studies like Dr. Cheraskin's give us some good guidelines for creating a vitamin supplementation program.

WHERE CAN YOU START?

The "minimum supernutrition" entry in the table that follows this chapter represents the best amount of a given vitamin for optimal results and minimal risk. If you are a smaller person with a low weight, or if your physical activity is somewhat below average, stay on the low side of the minimum supernutrition level. Your metabolism rate (the number of calories you consume daily, as discussed in Chapter 3) will also play a role: if it's high, you might use more vitamins; if low, try less. As we saw in Part II, you will need more vitamin

C if you smoke, are often under stress, and/or live in polluted air.

Vitamin supplementation should be done in stages. Start with a level close to your present state of nutrition and add increments. If you are not taking supplements now, a very conservative program to get you started would include the following: After breakfast take one multivitamin with minerals, some vitamin C with flavonoids (about 250 milligrams), and one calcium-magnesium (dolomite) tablet. After lunch: one vitamin C, and one B-complex. After supper: one vitamin C, one vitamin E (100 to 200 mg; be sure to read the precautions in the precaution table that follows this chapter), and one calcium-magnesium tablet. In case of diarrhea (which, for reasons unknown, can occur in some people), Spanora formulations, made from wild Spanish oranges, can usually solve the problem.

And Minerals

Vitamin advocates frequently make one major mistake; they forget about minerals and trace elements. There is no real difference between the two categories, except that some are used in larger amounts (calcium, magnesium, and phosphorus, for example) than others (such as iodine, iron, and zinc). A few are used only in traces—amounts so tiny that only very sensitive tests can detect their presence in the body—and it is this list of trace elements that is growing constantly. It currently includes copper, manganese, selenium, cobalt, chromium, and others.

Selenium now appears to be important in the prevention of heart disease and cancer, and it has been shown to be an essential nutrient in animals. Like vitamin E, selenium is an anti-oxidant. It may also prevent the "free radical" damage caused by adverse oxidation reactions. Drs. Raymond J.

Shamberger and Charles E. Willis of the Cleveland Clinic Foundation found that in areas where the amount of selenium was low in the surrounding soil, and therefore also low in the foods grown there, the heart attack rate was higher than in regions where the selenium concentration was higher. The same relationship was found for cancer: high selenium levels in foods were associated with lower cancer rates. Dr. John Martin of Colorado State University found that trace amounts of selenium can stimulate the immune system of test animals to perform up to 20 to 30 times more effectively than normal.

During food processing lots of selenium is lost from foods. A variety of good supplements are available from the Alacer Company (a combination of Vitamin E, selenium, and chromium), from Nutrition 21 (selenium-enriched brewer's yeast), from Cosvetics Laboratories (different types of selenium supplements), and from other companies.

Chromium is another trace mineral, and a deficiency of it has been linked with diabetes. We don't know yet exactly how this mechanism works, but we believe that vitamins and minerals combine to form enzyme systems that perform those metabolic reactions that are the basis for all cell functions. Even with all the needed vitamins present, nothing would work without the minerals.

The trace mineral zinc is found in several tissues of the body, especially in the prostate gland in men. It is now being investigated as a treatment for prostate trouble and for male sexual malfunctions.

Cobalt is the center atom of vitamin B_{12}, and there are many more trace minerals without which our cells could not perform normally.

Cadmium, lead, and mercury are the minerals we don't want in our systems, and they are difficult to get rid of. Chelation therapy, discussed in Chapter 11, is one method used in emergencies. The body itself sometimes uses the natural chemical leftovers from internal metabolic reactions to balance mineral levels, employing a natural chelation process to eliminate small amounts of unwanted minerals.

SOURCES OF TRACE MINERALS

Trace minerals are often found in the soil in extremely small quantities. When soil is used to grow crops for long periods of time without putting the minerals back into the soil, trace minerals become so low in concentration that foods grown there become deficient in them. Organic farming can prevent some of this depletion, but organic methods do not always supply all the other nutrients a plant needs. I would prefer to see a sensible combination of organic farming with mineral fertilizers, avoiding the use of pesticides as much as possible.

The best way to assure ourselves of superb and balanced nutrition would be to eat organically grown foods from all around the world. Since this is not possible, even small amounts of organically grown foods from your health-food store are helpful.

A WORD OF CAUTION

While we don't have to worry about excesses of most vitamins (within limits), the same does not hold for minerals. A slight excess won't do us any harm, but very large amounts, taken on a daily basis, can cause some medical problems.

For example, if a person uses iodized salt, takes a multivitamin with minerals that contains iodine, and additionally takes kelp (another source of iodine) and a mineral formulation, an excess of iodine could cause abnormal functioning of the thyroid. Large amounts of selenium (more than 1,000 micrograms per day) can be toxic; a supplement of 50 to 100 *micro*grams appears reasonable. Excessive quantities of zinc can cause metabolic disturbances; a supplement of 5 to 20 milligrams looks safe. Fluorine in just above average amounts will interfere with enzyme functions; that's why I oppose fluoridation of drinking water.

The average adult's calcium intake should be around 800 to 1,500 milligrams per day. The amount of phosphorus should not be more than twice the amount of calcium. Because of hormone differences, women usually need a little more calcium than men. The RDA for magnesium is 400 milligrams per day; the research literature on this mineral indicates that 400 to 600 milligrams per day is a reasonable range.

Since there is no reliable method for the layman to estimate mineral intakes, the best approach here would be to use the computerized Nutrition, Health, and Activity Profile recommended in Chapter 2. Once you know how much of each mineral you get from food sources, it is easier to design a supplementation program.

HAIR ANALYSIS

Mineral analysis of hair is another superb method that can tell a doctor about a patient's need for mineral supplementation, and it's also a good indicator of several metabolic disorders. While the blood or urine analysis can change from day to day, a hair analysis represents an average of minerals available to our cells. In one of our computer methods we combine a dietary analysis with a hair analysis; this combination allows the doctor to draw conclusions about possible malabsorption.

Table of Precautions

Vitamin A   Toxicity signs are dry, rough skin, yellowing of skin and eye whites, painful joint swellings, and nausea. Dosages above 30,000 IU a day for extended time periods should be carefully monitored by a doctor.

Vitamins B_1, $_2$, $_5$, $_6$, $_{12}$ Take a balanced supplement of B-complex vitamins, not just a partial selection. Reduce dosages if heart palpitations occur.

SUPERNUTRITION LEVELS FOR THE MAJOR VITAMINS

(*Important:* Be sure to read the Table of Precautions entry for each vitamin.)

Vitamin	RDA	---Supernutrition---		Toxicity Level	Remarks
		Starting Point	Maximum		
A	5,000 IU	10,000 IU	25–35,000 IU	75,000 IU	
B_1	1.5 mg	10–25 mg	100 mg	N.A.	
B_2	1.8 mg	10–25 mg	100 mg	N.A.	
B_3	20 mg	50 mg	250 mg– 3 grams	N.A.	
B_5	5–10 mg?	10–20 mg	100 mg	N.A.	RDA not yet established.
B_6	2 mg	10–25 mg	100 mg	N.A.	
B_{12}	3 mcg	5–10 mcg	100 mcg	N.A.	
C	45 mg	500–750 mg	4 grams	N.A.	
D	400 IU	400–500 IU	1,000 IU	40,000 IU	Toxicity level in children: 2,000 IU.
E	15 IU	200 IU	800 IU	N.A.	

Notes: "IU" means "international units;" "mg" means "milligrams;" "mcg" means "micrograms;" "N.A." means "not available"—the toxicity level is unknown. The figures in this table do not constitute recommendations; they simply represent vitamin levels for supernutrition proposed by Richard Passwater, Ph.D., in *Supernutrition for Healthy Hearts* (Dial Press), used with permission of the publisher.

Vitamin B$_3$ B$_3$ causes skin flushing if first taken in higher doses. Take this vitamin with other B-complex vitamins and reduce dosage if heart palpitations occur. Use with caution if you have glaucoma, severe diabetes, impaired liver function, or peptic ulcers.

Vitamin C   Reduce dosage if diarrhea occurs. The sodium ascorbate form (often found in chewable tablets) should not be taken by people on low salt (low sodium) diets. People taking anticoagulants should first consult their doctors. Vitamin C is a mild diuretic, but this is not a significant problem.

Vitamin D   People with heart disorders or kidney disease should use vitamin D with extra caution. Everyone should be aware of its possible toxicity.

Vitamin E   People with overactive thyroids, diabetes, high blood pressure, or rheumatic hearts should proceed cautiously. Start at 30 IUs per day for a month, then increase the daily dose by 30 IUs each month until a tolerance limit is reached.

Chapter 15

New Horizons in Aging Research

"With implanted cells, a clear revitalization, improved circulation, weight gain through better appetite in undernourished patients, and an overall improved mental performance, were observed in humans under clinical conditions."

Hermann Hoepke
Professor of Medicine
University of Heidelberg Medical
School
Heidelberg, Germany

The field of aging research, known as gerontology, is merging more and more with the field of preventive medicine and is rapidly yielding further clues about the processes that cause aging and the ways in which we can slow them down.

Unfortunately, two major factors are preventing the public from benefiting from researchers' efforts: a lack of funds and the Food and Drug Administration (which prevents doctors even from trying out new and successful treatments). If more money were available for staff and equipment to carry out the needed studies, many mysteries of the aging process would be cleared up within a few years. The trouble is that, even in cases where conclusive studies have been performed, the FDA does not allow public access to the latest methods. Any study performed in Europe is automatically rejected by the FDA, but that is just the beginning of this agency's exceedingly conservative standards and procedures for the approval of new drugs. And the sheer volume of FDA paperwork ensures that the approval process will, in many cases, take years longer than it should. In short, FDA regulations are so restrictive that in some areas they do more harm than good.

In other countries, where medical authorities are less hampered by conservative policies, many of the most recent advances in fighting aging are in practice. It is unfortunate that so many Americans are forced to spend millions of dollars seeking the most up-to-date medical attention abroad because they cannot find the treatments they need in the United States.

A short discussion of the treatments available elsewhere will enable interested readers to follow the development of these treatments in this country through newspaper and other media coverage, and will help you to decide whether to pursue such treatments for yourself. It will also put into perspective those therapies that have recently become available in the United States.

Cell Therapy

Cell therapy is a method, originally developed by Professor Paul Niehans in his private clinic in Switzerland just before World War II, in which cells from embryonic animal tissues are injected into the muscles of humans. These treatments are organ specific; that means cells from the heart strengthen the

196

heart of the treated person, cells from the liver revitalize liver functions, and so on. Various diseases are treated with this method, but it is also used to delay the manifestations of aging in general.

Even though the mechanisms of cell therapy revitalization are not yet 100 percent established, recent research in the medical field, using the most sophisticated equipment, has confirmed its effectiveness. I recently visited Germany and found that the conservative medical profession is still skeptical of this method, but then I also recognized that these people were not aware of the most recent work in this field.

Experiments since 1974 have established that the average lifespan of animals is increased with cell injections. On humans, cell injections have restored to normal the level of hormones in older people, established a resistance to cancer, and accelerated healing processes. Even the German government and private insurance companies have accepted this treatment for children with epilepsy, cerebral palsy, and mental retardation. Good results with cell injections were also reported by researchers in the United States.

WHERE IS CELL THERAPY PRACTICED?

Cell injections are accepted and practiced in many countries; Germany and Switzerland are the leaders. In Germany Dr. Siegfried Block is the director of the Privatsanatorium fuer Frischzellenbehandlung (D-8172 Lenggries, Obb.). Closer to home, Professor Ivan Poppov is the head of the Renaissance Clinic in Nassau in the Bahamas. In the United States the method is not accepted; doctors who try to practice it are harassed by the FDA.

THE LATEST RESEARCH RESULTS

In 1974 scientists from the Academy of Sciences in New York reported that cell injections can protect lungs from the effects of pollution. In another experiment Dr. A. Landsberger and Dr. C. Heym of the University of Heidelberg Medical School found that animals maintained good cell structures more successfully and for a longer time when they received cell injections. A sound cell structure and healthy cell functioning are equivalent to a delay in the overall aging process.

Dr. Katharina Scholz of Munich, Germany, reported exciting results after treating mongoloid children with a combination of conventional methods and cell injections. The cell injections gave clear improvements over the previously used methods. Professor Harry Feldmann in Geneva, Switzerland, used cell injections to treat mentally retarded children whose IQs ranged from 10 to 47. Over five years of cell therapy, their IQs improved by approximately 8.6 points per year.

Chapter 12 emphasized the importance of the immune system in the fight against cancer, and here again cell injections have been shown to be beneficial. The Cybila organization (Cytobiologische Laboratorien, Heidelberg, Germany) has developed a cell therapy formulation called Resistocell that stimulates immune responses and helps the body fight diseases. Professor of Medicine W. Zabel of Berchtesgaden, Germany, and Dr. Friedrich Blumenberg of the Strahlenklinik Janker in Bonn, Germany, published results of a human study in which conventional treatments were combined with cell injections. Definite improvements were observed in all cases, and a reversal of cancer growth was achieved in a few cancers, depending on the type.

The key, however, still lies in prevention. Staying away from as many factors as possible that have been associated with cancer formation is still your best bet. Even in individual cases, it is dangerous to say that cancer has been cured. If a cancer is successfully removed by surgery and if the patient makes drastic changes in his health habits and receives immunotherapy, then we can only say that the chance of survival is good; time then must show the effectiveness of the approach.

THE USE OF HUMAN CELLS

Since animal cells are somewhat different from human cells, using human cells for injections should yield better results. My conversations with doctors in this field lead me to believe that some of them have used human placenta cells, but nobody really wants to publicize this work. When results with human placenta cells were very good, and showed no negative side effects, Schwarzhaupt company in Germany went ahead and developed a formulation of human placenta cells. This formulation, besides being used for regular cell injections, has been found extremely helpful in accelerating healing processes in various tissues. Since only very small quantities are needed, these preparations also turned out to be quite inexpensive. Three ampules for cell injections cost only about $10. These preparations are not directly organ specific, but placenta cells have stimulated the functioning of the overall endocrine system by some other mechanism. Placenta cells are some of the most basic cells to all life processes, and there seem to be messenger compounds in these cells which trigger a whole chain of basic cell functions. The sad thing about it is that, if you want to take these injections, you have to travel long distances and spend a lot of money. Were they available in the United States, an administration of such a cell injection in your doctor's office as an outpatient would cost you only $30.

Nucleic Acid Therapy

Some researchers believe that the active ingredients in cell injections are the nucleic acids in the cells. There is DNA, the large molecule in the nucleus of every cell which contains all the basic information of the species. Cells also contain RNA acids that transport the information contained in the DNA throughout the cell. If we remove everything else from the animal cells and use the purified, organ specific nucleic acids as injections, we should see even more dramatic results. Such formulations are prepared by the Dyckerhoff Laboratorium in Cologne and are sold in Germany under the name "regeneresen." Brewer's yeast, too, is a good source for nucleic acids. (But don't start consuming huge amounts of brewer's yeast for this reason—you'll get a protein overdose!)

I have used small quantities of nucleic acids in animal experiments that yielded average life extensions of 30 to 50 percent. Present longevity studies indicate that, with higher concentrations, better results can be achieved. Supporting this view are some findings by German researchers who observed that nucleic acid injections stimulate the formation of interferon, a very important compound in immune reactions in our body. The best results, however, are achieved when nucleic acid injections are combined with other good health habits, including vitamins. These findings again support the Multi-Factorial Approach to slowing down aging.

Whenever a new preparation is used in medicine, our first concern should be to see if it causes any negative side effects. So far millions of nucleic acid injections have shown no harmful side effects. Indeed, the results are uniformly encouraging, even in cases where human patients were given nucleic acid dosages of several times the recommended amount and animals received dosages of up to 2,500 times the recommended amount.

In a study reported by Professor W. Gaus of the Dyckerhoff Laboratorium in Cologne, Germany, a formulation of nucleic acids from the inner ear improved a human subject's hearing capacity by several hundred percent. Only one to two injections were necessary every 1 to 2 months to maintain good hearing.

Three researchers at the Poliklinik in Hamburg-Eppendorf, Germany, found that nucleic acid injections accelerated the healing of fractures in animals. A personal experience of mine corroborates that finding: My mother, who had a very serious pelvis bone fracture at age 64, was given a 10 percent chance of ever walking again. She received nucleic acid injections made from several tissues and, within three years, was able to walk without a cane and return to her job in the family business.

Pros and Cons

The exact mechanism by which cell shots and nucleic acid injections operate is not known, and only continuing research will provide the answers. Until the exact mechanism for such an approach is established, many doctors hesitate to use it. I, too, would feel better if I knew exactly what happens in the body during these treatments, but the fact that the millions of treatments given to date (and that includes freeze-dried cell preparations made by Cybila) have caused no discernible negative side effects puts me somewhat at ease. As one doctor whose retarded daughter had been treated sucessfully with cell shots put it: "We are just so happy that this treatment worked on our daughter, I don't really care what the exact mechanism is."

MEANWHILE, BACK IN THE STATES

Some general nucleic acid formulations are available in the United States today, but when these products break down in the body they can release large amounts of uric acid. Too much of this substance can cause gout and other disorders. Therefore, anyone taking oral formulations of nucleic acids in relatively large amounts should have his or her uric acid level checked by a doctor and should follow a good vitamin supplementation program, since this can help the body control uric acid levels.

Concentrates

In 1951, researchers at the Children's Hospital Medical Center in Boston launched a study the results of which have had a considerable impact on American medicine. The disease under investigation was cystic fibrosis, a hereditary condition with symptoms which include severe digestive disorders and impaired functioning of the pancreas.

Subjects involved in the study were given a new formulation known as Viokase, a natural compound containing whole raw pancreas. The results were astonishing. Digestion was improved, often even normalized, and many other symptoms of cystic fibrosis also disappeared. The findings were subsequently confirmed by other medical authorities.

This was the start of a whole new line of products made from the organs or organ systems of animal tissue. Instead of treating certain diseases with drugs, doctors can now use a natural approach in which concentrates from specific organs are used to compensate for malfunctioning systems in the human body.

The two leading companies in this rapidly growing field are Nutri-Dyn in Skokie, Illinois, and Standard Process Laboratories in Milwaukee, Wisconsin. These companies manufacture a range of products from brain, pineal gland, heart, liver, and adrenal gland concentrates to formulations for older men and women that may well make hormone replacement therapy obsolete.

A SHORT SUMMARY OF THE ORGAN-CONCENTRATE MECHANISM

If we want to treat any malfunction in our body, we must first understand the functioning of the various organs. This is a highly technical subject, far too complicated for any reader without a background in the biological sciences. But in short, the ill or insufficient organ is studied, mechanisms for its functioning are established, and then materials from the equivalent organs of animals are used to bring the organ or organ system in question back to normal. The basic idea follows the same lines as the injections of organ specific nucleic acids or cell shots used in Europe.

The great advantage of extracts is that they allow a physician to treat organ disorders with a natural product instead of covering up the symptoms with drugs that, in many cases, don't get to the root of the problem. There are organ concentrates for nearly every organ problem, and they promise even more exciting results for the future.

A Reminder

The recent findings regarding cell shots, nucleic acid injections, and concentrates, exciting as they are, are not an open invitation to ignore the essential requirements for health as explained in Part II. It is still wisest to start your life-extension program by concentrating on the Seven Keys.

Chapter 16

The Center of Aging in the Brain

"We can trip the clock."

Dr. Marguerite Kay
National Institute on Aging
(Interviewed in *Fortune* magazine,
July, 1976)

"It's all in your head" is a timeworn phrase that has turned out to be accurate in many areas of medicine. Scientists are now finding that the saying applies to the aging process in ways that might never have been imagined a few decades ago. Researchers in the United States and elsewhere have found evidence that there is an "aging control center" in the brain that can be stimulated by certain foods and drugs to send the correct signals, sometimes called "youth signals," for the best possible functioning of the rest of the body. Experiments performed since 1965 also suggest that some diseases and mental disorders can be affected by the same substances.

This remarkable research has focused on the neuroendocrines (the part of the endocrine system in the brain), and on complex chemicals the body normally manufactures itself: "neurotransmitters," the chemicals nerve cells communicate with. Many of the research results are confusing and, at first glance, seem to contradict themselves. However, interpretations are not difficult if one views the evidence in light of my hypothesis on the functioning of this center of aging. Interpretations along these lines will also explain why it is possible to reverse male baldness patterns and why it will soon be possible to bring a woman back to the premenopausal state.

Neurotransmitters and the Aging Process

A precise discussion of the biochemistry of neurotransmitters would be far too complicated and not really necessary for an understanding of the basic principles involved. Since this is not a scientific paper, a few abbreviations and shortcuts will simplify the general approach and bring out the highlights.

Every time you think a thought, react to a situation, move a finger, or even breathe, million of microscopic nerve cells, "neurons," must communicate with each other. They do this by passing "neurotransmitters" back and forth at unbelievable speeds. The brain manufactures these essential chemicals itself, using amino acids from the protein in food as building blocks. There are several different neurotransmitters but, for simplicity's sake, let's just concentrate on the two most important ones, norepinephrine and serotonin. It is my hypothesis and interpretation of available research results that a minimum quantity of these neurotransmitters must be synthesized, and that a normal balance between them means perfect functioning or delayed aging of the entire body. The neurotransmitter serotonin is built from the amino acid tryptophane, and the amount of serotonin synthesized by the body depends very much on the availability of that amino acid from the blood stream. Likewise, the brain uses the amino acids tyrosine and phenylalanine to produce norepinephrine, the other major neurotransmitter.

Biochemists at some leading universities have recently discovered that by altering the body's balance of neurotransmitters, the aging process can be halted or reversed in laboratory animals. It appears that an imbalance of these neurotransmitters, with a decrease in norepinephrine or a relative increase in serotonin, means accelerated aging and/or mental disorders like depression.

At the University of California, Berkeley, Drs. Paul Segall and Harold Waitz in Professor Paola Timiras's research group found that when rats were put on a tryptophane-deficient diet for approximately half their lifespan, their entire growth and maturing process seemed to stop. When these animals were returned to a normal diet, they began to grow again, as if the time on the special diet had never passed at all. Rats 20 months old behaved as if they were half that age. They could even have offspring, a biological impossibility for normal rats that age.

What had happened? Since rats use tryptophane to manufacture serotonin (as do humans), the shortage of tryptophane and the relatively high amounts of tyrosine in the diet altered the rats' internal balance of neurotransmitters, apparently blocking the entire aging and maturing process. The implication of this discovery is staggering: Humans may someday be able to delay aging by eating foods with a specific amino acid ratio. WARNING: Do not reduce the tryptophane in your diet. It is an essential amino acid.

Dr. Caleb Finch, of the University of Southern California's Andrus Gerontology Center, has studied the aging control center in the brain extensively. His and others' results suggest that the hypothalamus and the pituitary, two glands in the front and middle section of the brain, also play a role in this aging control center.

Hormones: A First Look

Recent discoveries in baldness treatment give us a preliminary glimpse at the far-reaching effects of hormones in the body. Scientists have found that an imbalance of male and female hormones can bring on baldness in men, and have created shampoos and lotions that will balance the body's hormone levels to stimulate hair growth. (Two companies now market this product to doctors: Pilo-genic Research Associates, New York; and Cosvetics Laboratories, Atlanta.)

Additional research has shown, however, that the role of hormones goes far beyond the control of baldness.

Bringing a Woman back to the Premenopausal State?

It was always believed that, when a woman goes through menopause, aging of the endocrine system caused the decrease of hormone formation in the glands. In animals, menopause is equivalent to the point when female animals stop hormonal cycling. But Professor Joseph Meites at Michigan State University has demonstrated that certain hormone cycles in old female rats can be restarted by a mechanical stimulation of a specific area in the brain. Drs. M. Linnoila and R. Cooper at the Center for the Study of Aging, Duke University Medical Center, were able to bring back vaginal cycling in older animals with L-dopa and compounds normally used to treat depression. L-dopa, more commonly known for its role in the treatment of Parkinson's Disease, can be used by the body as an ingredient in norepinephrine. Any L-dopa in the system will affect the balance of neurotransmitters, which is apparently what happened in Linnoila and Cooper's test animals. This work suggests that, by affecting the center of aging in the brain, a woman could be brought back to the premenopausal state. Naturally, this would make estrogen-replacement therapy unnecessary.

Linnoila and Cooper's results also explain why, in earlier years, doctors observed a tremendous increase in the sex drive of Parkinson's disease patients who were given large amounts of L-dopa.

Procaine

Since the neurotransmitter balance plays such an important role in aging, it is not surprising that gerontologists have investigated numerous ways of affecting that balance. Joseph Hrachovec, a professor at USC's Andrus Gerontology Center, found that a compound called procaine can block the action of monoamineoxidase (MAO), an enzyme that destroys neurotransmitters, especially norepinephrine. When MAO is permitted to do this, the resulting neurotransmitter imbalance brings on aging.

Ana Aslan, a Rumanian medical professor and director of the Bucharest Geriatrics Institute, was the first (1940) to experiment with procaine's revitalizing effects. She was still studying the substance in 1974, when she described her most recent findings during the Miami Symposium on Theoretical Aspects of Aging. Many statesmen and celebrities have since received Dr. Aslan's procaine injections.

Since people would rather take a pill than an injection, the Schwarzhaupt Company in Germany developed an oral formulation known as KH–3. As usual, the United States is about the last country to allow this formulation to be sold. Efforts are being made to put it on the market here, now that numerous American scientists have confirmed research results published in the German medical literature as long as 20 years ago.

Neurotransmitters and Mental Disorders

In the December 1974 issue of *Psychology Today,* Drs. Jay Weiss, Howard Glazer, and Larissa Poherecky of Rockefeller University in New York presented some fascinating results of animal studies that showed a reduction of norepinephrine in cases of depression. Glazer and Poherecky were able to counteract depression by using substances that could inhibit MAOs destruction of norepinephrine.

MAO-inhibitors used in this country to treat depression have a large number of side effects. But researchers at leading medical schools have recently found that procaine can be used in the treatment of depression. The side effects of procaine are negligible compared to those of drugs presently used.

Procaine researchers have also observed impressive life extensions, a finding which demonstrates a definite connection between aging, mental disorders, and neurotransmitters.

The emphasis in my theory on the functioning of the control center in the brain is that there must be a "normal" balance of neurotransmitters. Future detailed research in this field will help us discover what "normal" is.

SCHIZOPHRENIA

This concept of a normal balance is nothing new. In the area of orthomolecular psychiatry ("ortho" means "correct" in Greek), a normal balance of molecules in the brain has been achieved with great success by using megavitamins, especially C, E, and niacin.

One psychiatrist at the 1975 convention of the International Academy of Preventive Medicine told me she used megavitamins to cure two patients with apparently hopeless cases of schizophrenia. Originally skeptical of megavitamins, she tried the technique only because the patients' parents had asked her to. With good nutrition and megavitamins, the illness began to subside almost immediately, and the two patients lead normal lives today.

Dr. Abram Hoffer wrote in the 1971 issue of *Schizophrenia*: "Any psychiatrist who begins with . . . 100 acute schizophrenics and follows the orthomolecular approach for a sufficient length of time, say three years, will find that 90% of his patients are well, the rest improved and none will be worse."

Despite this and other evidence in favor of the orthomolecular approach, the American Psychiatric Association has rejected it. APA studies of the subject seem to have been designed to prove orthomolecular therapy ineffective. For example, older schizophrenics were chosen for some APA experiments, almost guaranteeing that no positive results could be obtained. For a detailed discussion read Dr. Bernard Rimland's paper "Psychological Treatment Versus Megavitamin Therapy" in *Modern Therapies* (a Spectrum Book). People interested in seeking the services of a therapist can use *Modern Therapies* to determine what kind of approach they would feel most comfortable with and which would best suit their individual needs.

Hypoglycemia

For people who have hypoglycemia (low blood sugar), the balance between neurotransmitters plays a crucial role in mental health. In response to the low blood sugar level, the body tries to manufacture more glucose from amino acids already available. This conversion process consumes large amounts of most amino acids, including tyrosine and phenylalanine, but relatively little tryptophane. The unusually large proportion of tryptophane left over is transported to the brain, where it is converted into serotonin. The resulting imbalance between serotonin and norepinephrine can cause a person with hypoglycemia to become depressed and aggressive. In an article entitled "Food and Mood: What you eat may be what's eating you" (*Psychology Today,* December 1974), Dr. Brian Weiss discusses the relation of neurotransmitters to the aggressiveness of a tribe of Indians that had been found to be hypoglycemic.

The importance of a normal balance between neurotransmitters is underscored again by the finding that the body's norepinephrine level is highest during the day, and the serotonin level is highest at night when one sleeps. Psychiatrists have recently given people with insomnia small amounts of tryptophane, to help them sleep.

Longevity Studies

In my own longevity studies, I have used a variety of approaches to affect the balance between neurotransmitters in the brain. Some of the studies included procaine, vitamins, minerals, L-dopa, nucleic acid injections made from the hypothalamus and pituitary glands, amino acids, and other methods, but I achieved my best results by combining several of these approaches with exercise and good nutrition. I expect to lengthen the average lifespan of laboratory animals by at least 100 percent using this approach. Even though I have mentioned L-dopa, amino acids, and MAO inhibitors in these pages, I do not mean to imply that any readers should try to lengthen their lifespans by experimenting on themselves. Very careful research will tell us what the "normal" balance is. In one experiment I gave old animals 30 times the drug dosages I had used in a previous experiment. The animals livened up tremendously at first, but then they all died after only three days on this regimen.

It appeared they had burned the candle on both ends.

The discovery of neurotransmitters alone is not the solution to the larger question of aging. The "center of aging" in the brain is only part of the picture: Aging occurs everywhere in the body. Even if we can stimulate the center of aging to send signals to improve the functioning of specific organ systems, much will depend on the degree to which these systems have already been aged by bad health habits such as smoking, stress, and poor nutrition. The ability to stimulate the center of aging at age 70 or 80 will do little good for anyone whose health habits guarantee he'll die of cancer or heart disease at age 49.

Of course, more research must be done in this area before anyone can suggest diets to balance neurotransmitter levels in the body. But one piece of practical advice can already be given: Avoid distress, since it depletes the neurotransmitter norepinephrine.

The connection between hypoglycemia, schizophrenia, depression, aging, and the exotic chemicals that carry messages through the body may seem surprising. But as biochemical and medical research continues, many more surprises are no doubt in store, not the least of which might be a technique to reverse the aging process.

Part V

Success Through the Multi-Factorial Approach

A 63-year-old woman called the New School for Social Research recently and asked if she was too old for the crochet workshop. The registrar said that there were even older students there. The woman then asked if she could register for more than one course, and the answer was yes. Well then, she said, would the registrar also put her down for 'Aspects of Human Sexuality'?

The New York Times
May 24, 1973

Chapter 17

Assigning Priorities for Your Personal Anti-Aging Plan

> "In conclusion, it must be emphasized that senility is not an inevitable aspect of the aging process, but is a psychologic, biologic, social, and cultural phenomenon that is modified by intrapersonal, extrapersonal, and interpersonal attitudes."
>
> Alexander Simon, M.D.
> in *Aging: Prospects and Issues*

The previous chapters have presented a lot of material about numerous factors that contribute to the overall rate of aging. A logical reaction at this point would be "Great! But where should I start?"

When I discuss the Multi-Factorial Approach in public, people often pick out one or two points to work on and ignore others, reducing the effectiveness of the entire program. Giving specific advice for individuals is not easy because, as we have seen in the previous chapters, many anti-aging factors have to be considered in respect to others. What is important for one person might have a lower priority for another. And

215

on top of this comes the risk that 1 out of 1,000 persons might actually be negatively affected by a specific anti-aging measure because of his or her biochemical individuality.

To help you devise a program that will give the best possible results for your needs, this chapter ranks the anti-aging factors in order of decreasing priority. You can rate yourself in terms of each factor: E for excellent, R for reasonable, and U for unsatisfactory. Major changes are naturally up to you, with the help of your prevention-oriented doctor, but the general rule is to move ahead to points of lesser priority only when you have made provisions to correct existing problems in the more crucial areas.

Naturally, we would like every factor to check out as Excellent, but certain conditions make the acceptance of a Reasonable necessary. For example: the first five points deal with Super Nutrition, Normal Weight, Exercise, No Smoking and Alcohol Consumption. These are followed by factors of decreasing importance. It just wouldn't make any sense for a person who is overweight, doesn't eat right, and has no exercise program to worry about going to Europe and getting cell shots. So, the first unsatisfactory in the following checklist tells you exactly where to start your program.

Only when you have mastered points of highest priority will you be ready to deal with the successive points. Only by following the proper priorities can you expect the best results. If you decide not to follow this approach, you might observe some beneficial effects but the overall effectiveness of the Multi-Factorial Approach will be greatly decreased.

The Multi-Factorial Priority Scale

1). SUPERNUTRITION. As discussed in Chapter 3, life-expectancy and perfect functioning of the entire body

Excellent ☐
Reasonable ☐
Unsatisfactory ☐

can be enhanced by supplying our cells with the best possible nutrition. Research results indicate that the vast majority of people should make several changes in this area. Reevaluate your situation and, if you are uncertain about your intake of essential nutrients, have your dietary habits evaluated by a doctor or by a computer evaluation.

2). WEIGHT. Probably one of the most   Excellent ☐
important factors to be considered,   Reasonable ☐
proper weight is discussed in Chapters 3 Unsatisfactory ☐
and 4. If you have to lose weight, please do it right and don't use a crash diet or diet pills. If you are 5 to 10 percent over-weight, give yourself a "Reasonable"; more than that and you rate an "Unsatisfactory." Perfect weight is an "Excellent."

3). EXERCISE   As Chapter 4 indicates,   Excellent ☐
your regular schedule should include an   Reasonable ☐
endurance exercise like jogging or swim-   Unsatisfactory ☐
ming and a light muscle exercise for women or a heavier muscle exercise for men. If you are faithful about both kinds of exercise, you get an "Excellent"; if only one, "Reason-able"; if you have no exercise routine at all, your rating is "Unsatisfactory."

4). DON'T SMOKE   If you do, reading   Excellent ☐
Chapter 5 should convince you to cut   Reasonable ☐
down immediately, smoke only half the   Unsatisfactory ☐
cigarette, and plan to quit this health disaster soon. We know that antioxidants like vitamin C and E and the trace mineral selenium can protect us from the harmful effects of smoking. People who just can't quit should definitely take some of these compounds, but they shouldn't expect a 100 percent protec-tion from them.

Only nonsmokers who don't spend a lot of time in closed rooms with cigarette smokers get an "Excellent." If you smoke fewer than five cigarettes per day and/or spend time in cigarette-smoke-polluted air, give yourself a "Reasonable."

All you moderate-to-heavy smokers are definitely "Unsatisfactory."

5). ALCOHOL CONSUMPTION This factor is discussed in detail in Chapter 7. If you don't drink, or if you only have a few drinks at special occasions, or a beer or wine now and then, give yourself an "Excellent." Regular consumption of alcoholic beverages in small quantities gives you a "Reasonable." More than that is "Unsatisfactory."

Excellent ☐
Reasonable ☐
Unsatisfactory ☐

6). DISTRESS Chapter 8 explains that stress always exists in our lives, and only when it changes into distress, do we have to worry about it. No, or little, distress gives you an "Excellent." If distress often gets to you but you think you can handle it, this is a "Reasonable." If distress definitely affects your life for the worse, give yourself an "Unsatisfactory."

Excellent ☐
Reasonable ☐
Unsatisfactory ☐

7). VITAMIN AND MINERAL SUPPLEMENTATION As shown in Chapter 14, this factor depends very much on a person's nutrition and health habits and environment. The minimum requirement for most people is to take a good multivitamin with minerals, some vitamin C and E, and, depending on the outcome of a nutrition evaluation, possibly some calcium and magnesium and zinc. Stronger programs are necessary for people with hypoglycemia, diabetes, heart disease, depression, schizophrenia, and other serious diseases. If taking vitamin C causes diarrhea, cut back on the amount, or use a Spanora formulation made from wild Spanish oranges (available at health food stores). Alacer Company of Buena Park, Ca., makes a superb combination of Vitamin E, selenium, and chromium. Persons with diabetes, high blood pressure, a rheumatic heart, or an overactive thyroid should start with small doses and build up very slowly.

Excellent ☐
Reasonable ☐
Unsatisfactory ☐

8). REGULAR CHECKUPS, MONI-   Excellent ☐
TORING TRIGLYCERIDE AND CHO-   Reasonable ☐
LESTEROL LEVELS These should be Unsatisfactory ☐
done by a prevention-oriented doctor. If you don't know one,
write to one of the organizations listed in Chapter 10. One of
the first steps in any anti-aging programs should be to check
blood pressure and the levels of cholesterol, triglyceride, glucose, and uric acid in your blood. However, since so many
people rate so badly in the five highest-priority health factors,
an immediate complete blood analysis would only show that
changes are necessary in these areas. Therefore, you might
have a physical examination first, follow excellent health habits for a few weeks, and then have the blood analysis done. At
that point a blood analysis would probably confirm that you
are on the right track, and only minor adjustments might be
necessary.

Only if you have regular checkups with a prevention-oriented doctor, your cholesterol level is 190–170 or lower, and
your triglycerides are around 100 or lower, are you allowed
to give yourself an E. Values 10 to 15 points above these limits
will still qualify you for a "Reasonable," but everything else
is an "Unsatisfactory."

9). BIORHYTHM This science has   Excellent ☐
shown some dramatic results in the past   Reasonable ☐
few years and, although we do not yet Unsatisfactory ☐
completely understand why and how it works, no harm will
come by following it. It is the best tool we have in the area of
accident prevention. I have used it myself in controlling distress and in a weight-control program. Your own evaluation
of these areas will determine your rating. Award yourself an
"Excellent" if you plan to explore biorhythm further so you
can use it to fight distress. An accident-prone person who is
often under distress but neither uses nor plans to use biorhythm should definitely get an "Unsatisfactory."

219

10). AT PEACE WITH YOURSELF   Excellent ☐
Most of the points considered here deal   Reasonable ☐
with the biology and chemistry of aging   Unsatisfactory ☐
and the ways in which we can interfere with them. But a
prerequisite for the success of this approach is that a person's
head be straight. In a way, one has to develop a new philosophy and be willing to look at life with different eyes.

A major obstacle often standing in the way of making this
new approach work is the incapacity of people to face up to
themselves and admit that what they have been doing is not
good for them. When we have been smoking, drinking too
much, and getting no exercise for years, it is difficult to admit
to ourselves that we were wrong. In fact, for many people it
is almost impossible.

Misinformation on health is always readily available, and
too many people—even many scientists, who should know
better—are anxious to grab any distorted health story or easy-
to-use theory to justify their bad habits. I have heard the most
ridiculous excuses and justifications made by people who
wanted to continue abusing their bodies. A couple of the
more common lines: "My grandfather smoked all his life and
lived to be 90"; "When I get the urge to exercise, I sit down
and rest until the feeling goes away."

If a big-name university professor writes a scientifically
worthless book or article telling us that junk foods will improve our health 300 percent, you can be certain it will be
cited by people who refuse to admit their diet needs major
changes, or by people too lazy to make the changes they know
are necessary. Such books and articles are commonly filled
with twisted facts and statements the "authoritative" writers
wouldn't dare make in scientific publications. At the same
time, essential facts are likely to be omitted.

For example, take a recent article about regions whose

inhabitants chain smoke and drink heavily, yet live to uncommonly old ages. At one point, the writer of the article discussed a 104-year-old woman who smoked and drank, but doesn't mention the fact that she began smoking at age 69, that she smoked home-grown weeds and *not* tobacco, and that the other unusually old people did not smoke at all. Nor did the writer of the article report that the alcohol these people drank was home-brewed wine, in moderation, and that at the high altitude where they live, alcohol is literally exhaled through the lungs shortly after it is consumed. Despite all these omitted facts, one can be sure that people desperate to justify their smoking and excessive drinking will quote that article as gospel, never questioning for a moment its scientific validity or its unsound conclusions.

To improve your health and lengthen your life, you must be willing to accept the need for change. You must be able to approach the entire matter with the constructive attitude of someone who knows he or she has made mistakes and must make improvements, rather than someone anxious to cling to any excuse available. Without a positive attitude, the half-hearted efforts that are sure to result won't do you a bit of good.

So, when you see yourself continuing a bad health habit, be honest with yourself and find out why you are doing it, instead of justifying it with your own or somebody else's phony arguments. Then do something about it. If you feel you need professional help in achieving your goal, first evaluate the available therapies by reading *Modern Therapies,* by Virginia Binder, Arnold Binder, and Bernard Rimland (a Spectrum Book paperback).

Give yourself an "Excellent" for this item only if you can honestly say that you are willing and psychologically able to make a serious personal commitment to better health. You merit a "Reasonable" if you have a reasonably positive attitude about making the changes that need to be made, and you should give yourself an "Unsatisfactory" if, while reading this book, you have already tried to dream up excuses for not following one or more of the keys to a longer life.

11). CLEAN AIR AND WATER   As dis-   Excellent ☐
cussed in Chapter 6, if you live in highly   Reasonable ☐
polluted air, the only true solution is to   Unsatisfactory ☐
move out of the area. Because there are so many flagrant violations of our air pollution laws, because those laws are so poorly enforced, and because industrial polluters refuse to show concern for our health, the United States will not have truly clean air and water for many decades. We may never have an unpolluted environment. Too often, antipollution legislation is enacted, and we are happy about the regulations established under this legislation, but then we hear that industry has been given "another three years" or "another five years" to comply with the regulations. Now that this sorry performance has been repeated more times than anyone can count, is skepticism not warranted?

Whether pollution injures your health is not *entirely* beyond your control. If you drink a good well water, untouched by man, or a carbon- and micro-filtered water, and you live in a region with little or no air pollution, give yourself an "Excellent." If you breathe air with minor pollution, but take the right vitamins for antioxidant protection (see Chapter 5), give yourself a "Reasonable." Anything worse is an "Unsatisfactory."

12). PREPARING FOR FINANCIAL SE-   Excellent ☐
CURITY   As discussed in Chapter 9,   Reasonable ☐
you should start planning for retirement   Unsatisfactory ☐
at around age 20 or 25. You can give yourself an "Excellent" if you have a very good retirement program of your own or through your company, in addition to a savings plan. Social security plus a minor financial supplementation after retire-

222

ment gives you a "Reasonable," but social security alone is definitely an "Unsatisfactory."

Some Additional Anti-Aging Factors

Factors 1 through 8 are highly important, and "Unsatisfactory" ratings should be worked on immediately to achieve ratings of at least "Reasonable." As the next step, long-term plans should be made to change the "Reasonable" ratings to "Excellent," and only then should one attempt improvements in other areas.

Assigning a rating for factors 9 through 12 is often difficult because of a person's lifestyle and medical history. In addition to this, age and environment enter the picture. Some people might have found alternate methods of dealing with problems in these areas, and faulty conditions might be only temporary. Therefore, assigning a rating is left up to your good judgment.

Some additional factors have recently received attention in the health field, as well as in this book. Readers who have scored well so far may wish to consider more advanced anti-aging methods such as organ-specific concentrates, nucleic acids, and cell therapy (all in Chapter 15), procaine (Chapter 16), and hyperbaric oxygen (Chapter 13). Be sure to note any cautions given in those chapters.

And What Else Can You Do?

Relax and enjoy life. Following the Multi-Factorial Approach described in this book can give you at least 20 to 30 healthy and active years. In this extra time gerontologists will come up with more and more important ways to interfere with your aging process. You might even find it worthwhile to join the 500-club that was founded in Atlanta. But more about this in another book.

Notes

Chapter 1

RECOMMENDED TO GENERAL READERS

Degan, Charles. *Age Without Fear.* New York: Exposition Press, 1972.

ADDITIONAL REFERENCES

Strehler, Bernard. "Aging: Transcriptional and Translational Control Mechanisms and Their Alteration." Paper read at the 140th Meeting of the American Association for the Advancement of Science, 1974, at San Francisco.

Williams, Roger J. *Biochemical Individuality: The Basis for the Genetotrophic Concept.* New York: John Wiley & Sons, Inc., 1956.

Chapter 2

REFERENCES

Bjorksten, J.; Bloodworth, J.; and Buetow, R. "Enzymatic Lysis in Vitro of Hyalin Deposits in Human Kidney." *Journal of the American Geriatrics Society,* no. 4 (1972), pp. 148–150.

Breslow, Lester, and Belloc, Nedra. "Relationship of Physical Health Status and Health Practices." *Preventive Medicine,* no. 1 (1972), pp. 409–21.

Hayflick, Leonard. "Human Cells and Aging." *Scientific American,* no. 218 (1968), 19, 32–7

Kugler, Hans. "Slowing Down the Aging Process." *New Dynamics of Preventive Medicine,* vol. 4 (1976).

Packer, Lester, and Smith, James. "Extension of the in Vitro Lifespan of Human WI-38 Cells by Vitamin E." Paper read at the 4th Annual Meeting of the American Aging Association, 1974, at Los Angeles.

Chapter 3

RECOMMENDED TO GENERAL READERS

Brennan, R. O., and Mulligan, William C. *Nutrigenetics, New Concepts for Relieving Hypoglycemia: Case Studies.* New York: M. Evans and Company, 1976.

Cheraskin, E.; Ringsdorf, W. M.; and Brecher, Arline. *Psychodietetics.* New York: Stein and Day, 1974.
Fredericks, Carlton, and Goodman, Herman. *Low Blood Sugar and You.* New York: Grosset and Dunlap, 1976.
Hall, Ross Hume. *Food for Nought.* New York: Harper & Row, 1974.
Passwater, Richard. *Supernutrition for Healthy Hearts.* New York: The Dial Press, Inc., 1977.

ADDITIONAL REFERENCES
Burkitt, D.; Walker, A.; and Painter, N. "Effects of Dietary Fiber on Stools and Transit-Times, and its Role in the Causation of Disease." *Lancet,* no. 10 (1972), pp. 1408–11.
Cheraskin, E. "Influence of Nutrients on Behavior." Paper read at the Meeting of the International Academy of Preventive Medicine, 1975, at Los Angeles.
Cheraskin, E., and Ringsdorf, W. "Clinical Findings Before and After Dietary Counsel." *Geriatrics,* no. 27 (1972), pp. 121–26.
Lutwak, Leo. "Endocrine Changes With Age." Paper read at the 4th Annual Meeting of the American Aging Association, 1974, at Los Angeles.
Scrimshaw, Nevin S. "An Analysis of Past and Present Recommended Dietary Allowances for Protein in Health and Disease." *The New England Journal of Medicine,* no. 4 (1976), pp. 198–203.

Chapter 4

RECOMMENDED TO GENERAL READERS
DeVries, Herbert. *Vigor Regained.* New York: Prentice-Hall, 1974.
Emmerton, Bill. *Running for Your Life.* New York: Tower Press, 1971.
Rohe, Fred. *The Zen of Running.* New York: Random House, 1975.

ADDITIONAL REFERENCES
Anderson, James C. [Research studies performed at the Veterans Administration Hospital in Lexington, Kentucky. The results of these studies were released to the press in 1976 and were the subject of several articles.]
DeVries, Herbert. "Exercise Intensity Threshold for Improvement of Cardiovascular-Respiratory Function in Older Men." *Geriatrics,* no. 26 (1971), pp. 94–101.
"Prescription for Exercise for Older Men from Telemetered Exercise Heart Rate Date." *Geriatrics,* no. 26 (1971), pp. 102–111.
"What's a Joint Like That Doing in a Nice Person Like You?" *Prevention,* May 1974.
Gilmore, C. P. "Does Exercise Really Prolong Life?" *Reader's Digest,* July 1977, pp. 140–43. [Condensed from *The New York Times Magazine.*]
Morris, J.; Chase, S.; Adam, C.; Sirey, C.; Tech, B.; Epstein, L.; and Sheehan, D. "Vigorous Exercise in Leisure-Time and the Incidence of Coronary Heart Disease." *Lancet,* no. 1 (1973), pp. 333–38.

Chapter 5

RECOMMENDED TO GENERAL READERS

Clearing House on Smoking. [Request a list of their most recent books and pamphlets.] Atlanta, Georgia.

Reader's Digest. [Several articles on smoking have been published by this magazine. Your library should have back issues.]

Other organizations that will supply information on smoking and/or help you to quit smoking include: American Cancer Society, American Heart Association, American Lung Association, National Clearinghouse for Smoking and Health, National Tuberculosis and Respiratory Disease Association, Schick Center for the Control of Weight and Smoking, SmokEnders, and, Smoke Watchers.

ADDITIONAL REFERENCES

Auerbach, Oscar. Writings in *United Medical Laboratory News,* December 1971.

Callery, J. R. T. "Smoking: Harm to Your Children." *Science News,* December 14, 1974. *Lancet,* November 2, 1974.

Cheraskin, E. "Daily Tobacco Consumption and Lactic Dehydrogenase." *Journal of the International Academy of Preventive Medicine,* no. 1 (1976), pp. 10–14.

Cheraskin, E.; Ringsdorf, E.; and Medford, F. "Eating Habits of Smokers and Nonsmokers." *Journal of the International Academy of Preventive Medicine,* no. 2 (1975), pp. 9–18.

Russell, M. A., and Feyerabend, C. "Nicotine from Other Smokers." *Science News,* February 15, 1975. *Lancet,* January 25, 1975.

Science News. "Cigarette Gases and Tars Harmful." March 16, 1974.

Chapter 6

RECOMMENDED TO GENERAL READERS

Anderson, Bruce. *The Solar Home Book.* Harrisville, N.H.: Chesire Books, 1976.

Hodges, Laurent. *Environmental Pollution: An Introductory Textbook.* New York: Holt, Rinehart and Winston, Inc., 1973.

Montagu, Ashley. *The Endangered Environment.* New York: Mason and Lipscomb, 1974.

Murphy, John A. *The Homeowner's Energy Guide.* New York: T. Y. Crowell, 1977.

ADDITIONAL REFERENCES

Chemical and Engineering News. "Energy Executives: A New Breed of Managers." May 18, 1974.

Council of Environmental Quality. Report for 1975. [See also *Science News,* no. 107 (1975), p. 8.]

Harris, Robert, and Brecher, Edward. "Is the Water Safe to Drink?" *Consumer Report,* June and July of 1974, pp. 436–42 and 538–42.

International Joint Commission, Pollution of Lake Erie, Lake Ontario and the International Section of the St. Lawrence River. Washington, D. C.: Government Printing Office, 1970.

Los Angeles Times. "Harbor Oil Plan Raises Concerns." July 15, 1977.

National Enquirer. "Chlorinated Water Causes Cancer." [Detailed newspaper interviews with Drs. Robert Harris (associate director of the toxic chemicals program for the Environmental Defense Fund), Herbert Schwartz (Franklin Institute, Philadelphia), Michael Alavanja (Hunter College), and Nancy Reiches (Ohio State University Comprehensive Cancer Center).]

National Research Council. [1975 report on pollution emission standards.] [See also *Science News,* no. 107 (1975), p. 8.]

Sonstegard, Ron. "Cancerous Goiters and Tumors in Great Lake Fish." Paper read at the 20th Annual Conference on Great Lakes Research, 1977, at Ann Arbor, Michigan.

Wurster, C. "Chlorinated Hydrocarbon Insecticides and Avian Reproduction: How are they Related?" In *Chemical Fallout,* ed. M. Miller and G. Berg. Springfield, Illinois: Charles C. Thomas Publisher, 1972.

Chapter 7

RECOMMENDED TO GENERAL READERS

Bricklin, Mark. *The Practical Encyclopedia of Natural Healing.* Emmaus, Pa.: Rodale Press, Inc., 1976.

Chafetz, Morris. *Why Drinking Can Be Good For You.* New York: Stein and Day, 1976.

ADDITIONAL REFERENCES

American Business Man's Research Foundation. *Report on Alcohol.* Elmhurst, Illinois: 1971.

Badr, F., and Badr, Ragaa. "A Man's Drinking May Harm His Offspring." *Science News,* February 22, 1975. *Nature,* vol. 253 (1975), pp. 134–36.

Brady, Edwards, and Cluff, L. "Drugs and the Elderly." In *Drugs and the Elderly.* Los Angeles: Ethel Percy Andrus Gerontology Center (University of Southern California), 1973.

Chemical and Engineering News. "Drug Promotion Practices Scored at Hearing." March 18, 1974.

Cluff, Leighton; Smith, J.; and Seidl, L. "Studies in the Epidemiology of Adverse Drug Reactions." *Annals of Internal Medicine,* no. 65 (1966), pp. 629–40.

Diamond, John. *Collected Papers.* New York: Institute of Behavioral Kinesiology, 1977.

Iber, F. "In Alcoholism, the Liver Sets the Pace." *Nutrition Today,* no. 6 (1971), pp. 2–9.

Los Angeles Times. "FDA Urged to Open Drug Review Process." June 1, 1977.

Medical News. "High Carbohydrate Diet Affects Rat's Alcohol Intake." *Journal of the American Medical Association,* no. 6 (May 11, 1970), p. 976.

National Council on Alcoholism. "Criteria for the Diagnosis of Alcoholism." *American Journal of Psychiatry,* no. 129 (August 1972), pp. 127–35.

Offir, Carole Wade. "A Slavish Reliance on Drugs: Are We Pushers for Our Own Children? *Psychology Today,* no. 8 (December 1974), pp. 49–50.

Rodale, R. "Polluted Rats Turn to Drink." *Rodale's Health Bulletin,* no. 8 (July 25, 1970), p. 2.

Van Thiel, D.; Cagaler, H.; and Lester, R. "Ethanol Inhibition of Vitamin A Metabolism: Possible Mechanism for Sterility in Alcoholics." *Science,* no. 186 (1974), pp. 941–42.

Walker, Sidney. "Drugging the American Child: We're Too Cavalier About Hyperactivity." *Psychology Today,* December 1974, pp. 43–49.

Williams, Roger. "Alcoholism, Malnutrition of the Brain." *Let's Live,* February 1973.

Chapter 8

RECOMMENDED TO GENERAL READERS

Gittelson, Bernard. *Biorhythm: A Personal Science.* New York: Warner Books, 1977.

Selye, Hans. *Stress Without Distress.* New York: Signet Books, 1975.

Thommen, George. *Is This Your Day?* New York: Crown Publishers, Inc., 1973.

ADDITIONAL REFERENCES

Archer, J., and Blackman, D. "Prenatal Psychological Stress and Offspring Behavior in Rats and Mice." *Developmental Psychobiology,* no. 4 (1971), pp. 193–248.

Jenkins, David. "Behavior that Triggers Heart Attacks." *Science News,* no. 105 (1973), p. 402.

Selye, Hans. "Stress and Aging." *Journal of the American Geriatrics Society,* no. 18 (1970), pp. 669–80.

Timiras, P. *Developmental Physiology and Aging.* New York: The Macmillan Company, 1972.

Chapter 9

RECOMMENDED TO GENERAL READERS

Collins, Thomas. *The Complete Guide to Retirement.* Englewood Cliffs, New Jersey: Prentice-Hall, Inc., 1972.

Mendelson, Mary A. *Tender Loving Greed.* New York: Alfred A. Knopf, Inc., 1974.

ADDITIONAL REFERENCES

Department of Health, Education, and Welfare. *Your Social Security.* HEW Publication (SSA) 75–10035. Washington, D.C.: 1974.

Government Printing Office. *Retirement Income and Credit.* Government Publication 5018. Washington, D.C.: 1967.

Tax Benefits for Older Americans. Government Publication 5569. Washington, D.C.: 1967. [Ask for subsequent documents in this series.]

Los Angeles Times. "Medicaid Worst Rip-Off, Senate Panel is Told." November 18, 1976.

"Medicaid Pays Ineligibles $1 Billion, HEW Reports." April 30, 1977.

Malloy, Michael. "The Art of Retirement." *National Observer*, 1968.

Shore, Warren. "Social Security—The Great Ripoff?" *Chicago Today*, April 29–May 3, 1974. [Five-part series.]

Chapter 10

RECOMMENDED TO GENERAL READERS

Illich, Ivan. *Medical Nemesis.* New York: Pantheon, 1976.

Selye, Hans. *The Stress of Life.* New York: McGraw-Hill Publishing Co., Inc., 1956.

ADDITIONAL REFERENCES

Brennan, R. O. "IAPM Objectives: A Positive Renewal." *Journal of the International Academy of Preventive Medicine*, no. 1 (1976), pp. 5–9.

Cordas, Steven. "Nutrition and Ecology." *Journal of the International Academy of Preventive Medicine*, no. 2 (1976), pp. 5–7.

Fredericks, Carlton. "The 'Ouch!' of Prevention." *Journal of the International Academy of Preventive Medicine*, no. 3 (1975), pp. 5–7.

Los Angeles Times. "Bill of Health, Patient's Bad Habits Push Costs Higher." July 26, 1977.

Pomeroy, Leon. "From the Editor's Desk." *Journal of the International Academy of Preventive Medicine*, no. 2 (1976), pp. 5–8.

Chapter 11

RECOMMENDED TO GENERAL READERS

Harper, Harold, and Culbert, M. *How to Beat the Killer Diseases.* New Rochelle, N.Y.: Arlington House, 1978.

Passwater, Richard. *Supernutrition for Healthy Hearts.* New York: The Dial Press, Inc., 1977.

ADDITIONAL REFERENCES

Brown, Michael, and Goldstein, Joseph. "Inheritance and High Cholesterol." *Science News*, no. 106 (1974), p. 22.

Crawford, M.; Clayton, D.; and Morris, J.; Cardiovascular Disease in Hard and Soft Water Areas. *Lancet*, no. 1 (1973), pp. 613–14.

DeVries, Herbert. "Exercise Intensity Threshold for Improvement of Cardiovascular Respiratory Function in Older Men." *Geriatrics*, no. 26 (1971), pp. 94–101.

Dahl, K. Untitled lecture given at Georgetown University Medical School, April 1974.

Ginter, Emil. "Vitamin C and Cholesterol." *Science*, February 16, 1974.

Glueck, Charles. "Does It All Start Here?" In *Atherosclerosis.* New York: MEDCOM, Inc., 1974.

Harper, Harold, and Gordon, Garry. *Reprints of Medical Literature on Chelation Therapy.* American Academy of Medical Preventics, 11311 Camarillo Street, North Hollywood, California 91602.

Housley, E., and McFadyen, I. "Vitamin E in Intermittent Claudication." *Lancet*, no. 1 (1974), p. 468.

Jick, H.; Miettinen, O.; Neff, R.; Shapiro, S.; Heinonen, O.; and Slone, D. Coffee and Myocardial Infarction. *New England Journal of Medicine,* no. 289 (1973), pp. 63–67.
Keys, Ancel. "Coronary Heart Disease—The Global Picture." *Artherosclerosis,* no. 22 (1975), pp. 149–92.
Kugler, Hans J. "Prevention of Diseases of the Arteries: A Basic Requirement for Extending the Human Life Span." Paper read at the Meeting of the American Academy of Medical Preventics, 1975, at Los Angeles.
Lown, B.; Verrier, R.; and Corbalan, R. "Psychologic Stress and Threshold for Repetitive Ventricular Response." *Science,* no. 182 (1973), pp. 834–36.
Morris, J. N. "Physical Activity and Heart Disease Prevention." *Lancet,* no. 1 (1973), p. 333.
Mumma, R. "Dissolution of Cholesterol from Animal Arteries by Ascorbic Acid and Derivatives." Paper read at the Meeting of the Federation of American Societies for Experimental Biology, 1971, at Philadelphia.
Passwater, Richard. "Dietary Cholesterol, Is it Related to Serum Cholesterol and Heart Disease?" *American Laboratory,* September 1972.
Pritikin, Nathan. "Diet and Exercise as a Total Therapeutic Regimen for the Rehabilitation of Patients with Severe Peripheral Vascular Disease." Paper read at the Meeting of the International Academy of Preventive Medicine, 1976, at Denver. Also read at the 52nd Annual Congress of Rehabilitation Medicine, 1975, at Atlanta, Georgia.
Stamler, Jeremiah. "The Statistics Do Speak: Listen." In *Atherosclerosis,* New York: MEDCOM, Inc., 1974.
Yacowitz, Hal. "Beneficial Effects of High Levels of Vitamin E in Improving Blood Circulation in Humans." *Feedstuffs,* June 2, 1975, p. 26.

Chapter 12

REFERENCES
Arehart Treichel, Joan. "Cancer and the Body's Defense System." *Science News,* June 23, 1973.
Hoover, Robert; Mason, Thomas; McKay, Frank; and Fraumeni, Joseph. "Cancer by County: New Resource for Etiologic Clues." *Science,* September 19, 1975.
Medical World News. "Diet's Role in Carcinogenesis." February 25, 1972.
Mirvish, S.; Wallcave, L.; Eagen, M.; and Shubik, P. "Vitamin C Blocks Carcinogens." *Science News,* July 22, 1972.
Passwater, Richard. "Cancer New Directions.: *American Laboratory,* June 1973.
Pinckney, E. R., and Pinckney, Cathey. *The Cholesterol Controversy.* Los Angeles: Sherbourne Press, 1973.
Rauscher, Frank. "Breast Surgery Controversy." *Science News,* no. 106 (1974), p. 232.
Renner, H. "Onko fetale Antigene und Tumor-Immuntherapie." *Fortschritte Der Medizin,* no. 5 (1974), pp. 175–78.
Shamberger, R.; Baughman, F.; Kalchert, S.; Willis, C.; and Hoffman, G.

"Carcinogen-Induced Chromosomal Breakage Decreased by Antioxidants." *Proceedings of the National Academy of Science,* no. 70 (1973), pp. 1461–63.
Sullivan, Henry. "Bronchogenic Carcinoma: The True Story." *Geriatrics,* March 1973, pp. 140–42.
Tappel, A. I. *Pathological Aspects of Cell Membrances.* New York: Academic Press, 1961.

Chapter 13

REFERENCES
Hare, Edward; Price, John; and Slater, Eliot. "Schizophrenia in Winter." *Science News,* no. 105 (1973), p. 402. *British Journal of Psychiatry,* vol. 124, 1973.
Hart, George B. "Hyperbaric Oxygen in Cardiovascular Disease—Acute and Chronic." Paper read at the Meeting of the American Academy of Medical Preventics, 1976, at Kansas City, Missouri.
Hoffer, A., and Osmond, H. *How to Live with Schizophrenia.* New Hyde Park, New York: University Books, Inc., 1974.
Hare, Edward; Price, John; and Slater, Eliot. "Mental Disorder and Season of Birth: A National Sample Compared with the General Population." *British Medical Journal,* no. 124 (1974), pp. 81–86.
Pfeiffer, C.; Ward, J.; El-Meligi, M.; and Cott, A. *The Schizophrenias: Yours and Mine.* New York: Pyramid Books, 1970.
Schachter, Michael. "Nutrition in Orthomolecular Psychiatry." Paper read at the Meeting of the Academy of Orthomolecular Psychiatry, 1976, at Kansas City, Missouri.
Wisniewski, Henryk, and Terry, Robert. "Aging in the Nervous System." Paper read at the 104th Meeting of the American Association for the Advancement of Science, 1974, at San Francisco.
Wunderlich, Ray. "Paranoid Schizophrenia as a Manifestation of Metabolic Derangement: Successful Management by Metabolic Therapy." *Journal of the International Academy of Preventive Medicine,* no. 1 (1976), pp. 21–36.

Chapter 14

RECOMMENDED TO GENERAL READERS
Rosenberg, Harold, and Feldzaman, A. N. *The Doctor's Book of Vitamin Therapy.* New York: G. P. Putnam's Sons, 1974.
Stone, Irwin. *The Healing Factor: Vitamin C Against Disease.* New York: Grosset & Dunlap, Inc., 1972.

ADDITIONAL REFERENCES
Cheraskin, E.; Ringsdorf, W.; and Medford, F. "The Ideal Daily Vitamin A Intake." *International Journal for Vitamin Research,* no. 1 (1976), pp. 11–13.
"The Ideal Daily Niacin Intake." *International Journal for Vitamin Research,* no. 1 (1976), pp. 58–60.
Coulehan, John; Reisinger, Keith; Rogers, Kenneth; and Bradley, Daniel.

"Vitamin C Prophylaxis in a Boarding School." *New England Journal of Medicine*, January 3, 1974, pp. 6–9.

Klenner, F. R. "Significance of High Daily Intake of Ascorbic Acid in Preventive Medicine." *Journal of the International Academy of Preventive Medicine*, no. 1 (1974), pp. 45–69.

Maugh, Thomas. "Vitamin A: Potential Protection from Carcinogens." *Science*, no. 186 (1974), p. 1198.

Passwater, Richard. "B-15 May Be As Valuable As Vitamin E." *Let's Live*, January, February 1976.

Rudolph, Charles J. "Trace Element Patterning in Degenerative Diseases. *Journal of the International Academy of Preventive Medicine*, vol. 4 (July 1977), pp. 9–31.

Yew, Man-Li. "Vitamin C and Wound Healing." *Proceedings of the National Academy of Sciences*, April 1973. *Science News*, no. 103 (1973), p. 290.

Chapter 15

REFERENCES

Bethge, J. F., and Nagel, K. H. "Versuche zur Verkuerzung der Frakturheilzeit." *Langenbecks Archiv fuer Klinische Chirurgie*, no. 333 (1973), pp. 153–64.

Fredman, Steven; and Burger, Robert. *Forbidden Cures: How the FDA Surpresses Drugs We Need.* New York: Stein and Day, 1976.

Gaus, W., and Isnel, A. *Physikalische Medizin und Rehabilitation*, vol. 5, May 1970.

Feldman, Harry. "Vergleichende Laengsschnitt-Studie ueber die verschiedenen medikamentoesen Behandlungen der geistigen Retardierung." *Die Zelltherapie*, no. 41 (1974), pp. 85–104.

Hoepke, Hermann. "Die Wissenschaftliche Grundlage der Zelltherapie" In *Zur Wirkungsweise Unspecifischer Heilgergahren*. Hippokrates Verlag, 1972.

Odens, Max. "Prolongation of the Life Span in Rates with RNA and DNA Injections." *Journal of the American Geriatrics Society*, no. 10 (1973), pp. 450–51.

Orzechowski, Georg. "Moleculare Biologie." *Zeitschrift fuer Therapie*, no. 6 (1974), pp. 321–35.

Schmid, F. "Therapeutischer Nihilismus beim Mongolismus ist heute nicht mehr zu verantworten. *Medical Tribune* [German edition], no. 10, March 8, 1974.

Scholz, Katharina. "Erfahrungen mit der Zelltherapie bei mongoloiden Kindern." *Die Zelltherapie*, no. 41 (1974), pp. 58–74.

Schwachman, Harry; Redmond, Aileen; and Khaw, Kon-Taik. "Studies in Cystic Fibrosis." *Pediatrics*, no. 46 (1970), pp. 335–43.

Toskes, R. "Pancreatic Supplements in the Control of Cystic Fibrosis." *New England Journal of Medicine*, no. 284 (1971), pp. 627–32.

Toskes, Phillip; Hansell, John; Cerda, James; and Deren, Julius. "Vitamin B-12 Malabsorption in Chronic Pancreatic Insufficienty." *New England Journal of Medicine*, no. 284 (1973), pp. 627–32.

Von Langendorff, Langer. "Schutzwirkung der Zelltherapie gegen emphysembedingte Lungendegeneration." *Die Zelltherapie,* no. 41 (1974), pp. 3–12.

Chapter 16

RECOMMENDED TO GENERAL READERS

Binder, Virginia; Binder, Arnold; and Rimland, Bernard. *Modern Therapies.* Englewood Cliffs, New Jersey: Spectrum Books, 1976.

ADDITIONAL REFERENCES

Cohen, Sidney, and Ditman, Keith. "Gerovital H3 in the Treatment of the Depressed Aging Patient." *Psychosomatics,* no. 14 (1974), pp. 15–19.

Hrachovec, J. "MAO Inhibition by Procaine." Paper read at the 26th Annual Meeting of the Gerontological Society, 1973, at Miami Beach, Florida.

Kugler, Hans. "Slowing Down the Aging Process: Recognizing the True Causes of Aging." Paper read at the Life Extension and the Control of Aging Conference, Wholistic Health & Nutrition Institute, 1977, at Mill Valley, California.

Latham, Keith. "The Neuropathology of Aging." Paper read at the Life Extension and the Control of Aging Conference, Wholistic Health & Nutrition Institute, 1977, at Mill Valley, California.

Linnoila, M., and Cooper, R. "Reinstatement of Vaginal Cycles in Aged Non-cycling Female Rats." Paper read at the Fall Meeting of the Gerontological Society, 1975, at Duke University.

MacFarlane, David, and Besbris, Howard. "Procaine (Gerovital H3) Therapy: Mechanism of Inhibition of Monoamine Oxidase." *Journal of the American Geriatrics Society,* no. 8 (1974), pp. 365–71.

Mock, A. "Die Psychische Effizienz eines Geriatrikums." *Aerztliche Praxis,* no. 22 (1970), p. 1999.

Pakesch, E. "Die Behandlung und Prophylaxe arteriosclerotischer Geistes-stoerung." *Wiener Klinische Wochenschrift,* no. 82 (1970), p. 211.

Segall, Paul, and Waitz, Harold. "Long term Tryptophane Deficiency and Aging in the Rat." Paper read at the 4th Annual Meeting of the American Aging Association, 1974, Los Angeles.

Weiss, Jay; Glazer, Howard; and Poherecky, Larissa. "Neurotransmitters and Helplessness: A Chemical Bridge to Depression?" *Psychology Today,* no. 8 (1974), pp. 58–60.

Index

Academy of Orthomolecular Psychiatry, 135
Accidents
biorhythm and, 112–13
See also Automobile accidents
Activated carbon (charcoal), 85, 86
Additives, 39
average American's consumption
of, 40
cancer and, 164–65
in longevity quiz, 14
Adler, W. H., 158
Advertising, cigarette, 67–68
Aerosol sprays, 103
Aging, 20–32
brain's control center for, 3, 23–
25, 204–12
combination theory on, 25, 28–
30, 172

research into, 3, 195–212
animal model, 25–28
See also Cell therapy; Nucleic-
acid therapy; Organ-specific
concentrates; Procaine therapy
reversal of, 30–32
sickness and, 131
stress and, 107–8
AHH enzyme, 163
Air pollution, 73–80
body damage from, 74
how to reduce, 77–80
longevity and, 73
in longevity quiz, 16
from oil terminals, 76–77, 163–
64
in priority scale, 222
smoking and, 71